COMPLEX REGIONAL PAIN SYNDROME(CRPS):

LEARNING ABOUT THE DIFFERENT ASPECTS OF A PAINFUL SYNDROME

Volume-VI

Eric M. Phillips

COMPLEX REGIONAL PAIN SYNDROME (CRPS):

LEARNING ABOUT THE DIFFERENT ASPECTS OF A PAINFUL SYNDROME
Volume-VI

Copyright © 2024 by Eric M. Phillips

First edition, 2024 – Volume-VI

ISBN: 9798332241031

Other books published by the author:

Complex Regional Pain Syndrome (CRPS): Patients' Perspective of Living in Chronic Pain: Volume 1

Complex Regional Pain Syndrome (CRPS): Patients' Perspective of Living in Chronic Pain: Volume 1-Picture eBook

Don't Diet: Change Your Eating Habits - Proper Eating for Good Health

Complex Regional Pain Syndrome (CRPS): Patients' Perspective of Living in Chronic Pain: Volume II

Complex Regional Pain Syndrome (CRPS): Patients' Picture eBook Guide: Volume II

What is CRPS? A Helpful Guide to Teach Children About Complex Regional Pain Syndrome (CRPS): Volume III

Complex Regional Pain Syndrome (CRPS) and Amputation: A Patients' Picture eBook Guide: Volume III

Complex Regional Pain Syndrome (CRPS) and Amputation: A Difficult Decision to Make: Volume IV

Complex Regional Pain Syndrome (CRPS): Patients' Picture eBook Guide: Volume IV

Complex Regional Pain Syndrome (CRPS): Patients' Perspective of Living in Chronic Pain: Volume V

Complex Regional Pain Syndrome (CRPS): Patients' Perspective of Living in Chronic Pain: Volume VI

Complex Regional Pain Syndrome (CRPS): Patients' Perspective of Living in Chronic Pain: Volume VII

Complex Regional Pain Syndrome (CRPS): Learning About The Different Aspects of a Painful Syndrome: Volume I

Complex Regional Pain Syndrome (CRPS): Learning About The Different Aspects of a Painful Syndrome: Volume II

Complex Regional Pain Syndrome (CRPS): Learning About The Different Aspects of a Painful Syndrome: Volume III

Complex Regional Pain Syndrome (CRPS): Learning About The Different Aspects of a Painful Syndrome: Volume IV

Complex Regional Pain Syndrome (CRPS): Learning About The Different Aspects of a Painful Syndrome: Volume V

Learning Cursive is Fun-A Step-by Step Writing Guide for Beginners

Handwriting Practice Papers- 100 Pages

Handwriting Practice Papers- 200 Pages

Handwriting Practice Papers- 300 Pages

ABC's and 123's Tracing Guide Book: A Step-by-Step Tracing Guide for Children Ages 3-6. Includes A 26-Page Coloring Book

Cursive Handwriting Practice Book for Teens- 200 Pages

Addition and Subtraction Practice Workbook-For Grades 1-2

Multiplication and Division Practice Workbook-For Grades 3-5

What Time Is It Now: A Helpful Guide to Help Kids Tell Time

DEDICATION

To my loving parents, Janet, and my late father Leonard (Lenny), and my two older brothers Michael and Keith, and their families for all their love, and support.

To my beautiful and supportive wife Mercedes, her three children, Raymond, Serena, Stephanie, and her grandson Damian.

To my best friends Mike I., and Jim H., for your friendship and support.

To my mentor, teacher, and greatest friend the late Doctor Hooshang Hooshmand.

To all CRPS patients worldwide. Keep being strong!

To all my relatives from Ukraine and to all the Ukrainian people who are dealing with this current senseless crisis in Ukraine.

"Slava Ukraini!" (Glory to Ukraine!)

IN MEMORIAM

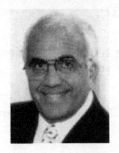

Doctor Hooshang Hooshmand
1934-2019

Doctor Hooshang Hooshmand, dedicated his life to medicine (Neurology), teaching, and caring for his patients for over 40-years.

He had a special interest in the management of Reflex Sympathetic Dystrophy (RSD), and other neurological conditions such as Multiple Sclerosis (MS), Epilepsy, and Electrical Injuries.

- He had such a grand passion for writing on many medical topics like RSD, Cerebrospinal Fluid Pressure, Topographic Brain Mapping, Electrical Injuries, Thermography, and including this book on Diet.

- He made many landmark contributions to medicine over his 40-year career.

- First to use Klonopin (clonazepam) for treatment of epilepsy in the United States. (1968-1973).

- First to report beneficial effects of Adrenocorticotropic hormone (ACTH) in the stimulation of endorphins for treatment of chronic pain (1987).

- First to standardize technical requirements of topographic brain mapping (1987 and 1989).

- First to report the CNS damage of electrical injuries diagnosed by evoked potentials (1989).

- First to recommend treatment of neurosyphilis with mega-doses (over 20 million u) Penicillin (1972): later adopted by the World Health Organization in 1972.

- First to report the mechanism of action of Decadron (dexamethasone) in treatment of increased intracranial pressure (1969).

- First Textbook on Reflex Sympathetic Dystrophy (RSD) (1993).

Doctor Hooshmand had a great philosophy and understanding of medicine. He was ahead of his time and always looked outside of the box with his approach to treating such conditions as RSD-CRPS.

His philosophy on treating RSD-CRPS was to approach it in a multidisciplinary fashion with the use of proper non-addictive medications, proper nerve blocks, proper physical therapy, having a proper diet, and avoiding unnecessary surgeries.

He was a great advocate for his patients. He truly loved helping his patients to receive the proper treatment and care they needed. He always tried giving them a better quality of life from the pain they were suffering. He always treated his patients with compassion and with the utmost respect.

He had so much compassion for life, medicine, and helping his patients. If a patient could not afford treatment or a test they needed to help with a diagnosis, he would treat the patient free of charge. Treating a patient for free in this day and age is unheard of. This was how Doctor Hooshmand was. He was so generous with his time, with his willingness to help others, and sharing his vast knowledge of medicine and CRPS. He was remarkable in the way he wanted to help others.

One of my favorite Doctor Hooshmand lines he would say to people (mostly doctors) who were attending his RSD-CRPS lectures was, "Do you know the difference between God and a Doctor? The answer is: God does not think he is a doctor, but most doctors think they are God's." The first time I heard him say this was in front of a group of doctors. It blew my mind away, by what he had said in front of these doctors. To be honest, he was 100% right in what he was saying.

I have been so fortunate to have known and worked with Doctor Hooshmand for over 25-years. He was the greatest mentor and friend anyone could ever ask for. I cannot thank him enough for sharing his incredible knowledge with me and the world.

He has now left us for his next journey in life, but he has left a lasting impression on so many of us that we can never repay him back.

His life's work through his research and his writings will help many people for generations to come.

Eric M. Phillips

QUOTES BY: DOCTOR HOOSHANG HOOSHMAND

I want to share some impactful and inspiring quotes written by my mentor and best friend, the late Doctor Hooshang Hooshmand.

To all CRPS Patients: "Remember, CRPS is not all in your head." It is all over your body. It starts from one extremity or one part of the body, and if not properly treated, it spreads to the other parts of the body. Do not let anybody convince you to be treated exclusively by a psychiatrist or to learn to live with your pain. Just remember you are not crazy. The pain of CRPS is enough to drive anybody out of their mind, but what I admire is the fact that CRPS patients still keep their sanity. H. Hooshmand, M.D.

Reflex sympathetic dystrophy (RSD) is the most unpleasant and uncomfortable form of chronic pain. It is the extreme prototype of disabling chronic pain. H. Hooshmand, M.D.

A Doctor's Explanation: "I cannot treat what I cannot see" An old medical phrase provides a contrast: "The Brain cannot conceive when the eye cannot see." H. Hooshmand, M.D.

As my mother said: "Do not cut what you can untie." H. Hooshmand, M.D.

TABLE OF CONTENTS

PREFACE..1
Eric M. Phillips

INTRODUCTION 3
Eric M. Phillips

CHAPTER 1
THE DIFFERENCE BETWEEN COMPLEX REGIONAL PAIN SYNDROME
(CRPS), FIBROMYALGIA(FM), AND MYOFASCIAL SYNDROME(MFS)........5
Eric M. Phillips

CHAPTER 2
COMPLICATIONS CAUSED BY NERVE BLOCKS IN
COMPLEX REGIONAL PAIN SYNDROME (CRPS)......................................22
Eric M. Phillips

CHAPTER 3
TREATMENT WITH ICE CAN CAUSE COMPLICATIONS IN
COMPLEX REGIONAL PAIN SYNDROME (CRPS).....................................44
Eric M. Phillips

CHAPTER 4
MULTIPLE LIMB AND TOTAL BODY COMPLEX REGIONAL PAIN
SYNDROME (CRPS)..60
Eric M. Phillips

CHAPTER 5
COMPLEX REGIONAL PAIN SYNDROME (CRPS) AND PREGNANCY.........83
Eric M. Phillips

CHAPTER 6
ENDOCRINE SYSTEM DYSFUNCTION(ESD) IN
COMPLEX REGIONAL PAIN SYNDROME (CRPS)................................94
Eric M. Phillips

CHAPTER 7
ELECTRIC SHOCK PAIN(ESP) IN
COMPLEX REGIONAL PAIN SYNDROME (CRPS)................................102
Eric M. Phillips

CHAPTER 8
PARESIS COMPLICATIONS IN
COMPLEX REGIONAL PAIN SYNDROME (CRPS) 113
Eric M. Phillips

CHAPTER 9
INTERNAL ORGAN COMPLICATIONS IN
COMPLEX REGIONAL PAIN SYNDROME (CRPS)................................121
Eric M. Phillips

CHAPTER 10
THE NAME CHANGE: WHAT SHOULD WE CALL IT? CAUSALGIA, RSD,
CRPS, OR SOMETHING NEW?..132
Eric M. Phillips

CRPS INFORMATION RESOURCE PAGE 156

PREFACE

For over 34-years, I have worked in the CRPS community to help advocate on behalf of other CRPS patients. Because I have lived with CRPS for over 38-years, and have been an amputee going on 16-years this August, I am very familiar with the struggles and pain that CRPS patients endure.

During the past 38-years of living with CRPS, I feel that the biggest downfall for most CRPS patients is the lack of understanding of the disease by the medical community and public.

I believe that providing education and raising awareness on CRPS is crucial to ensure patients receive proper care and a better quality of life.

Over the years, I have been fortunate and blessed to have work with my mentor and best friend, the late Doctor Hooshang Hooshmand, and my good friend, Doctor Alaa Abd-Elsayed. It has been an honor to work with and learn from these two prominent physicians. Over the past several decades, I have collaborated with these two remarkable physicians on many important CRPS projects to help bring more awareness and education about CRPS.

I felt writing this sixth book about the different aspects of CRPS would help educate the public, as well as the medical community, about the severity and reality of this disease, which affects millions of people worldwide.

Moreover, to help others understand how patients live and cope with this unrelenting painful disease. CRPS patients are only looking for some form of pain relief, and a better quality of life.

We have to remember when it comes to treating CRPS, physicians should look outside of the box to understand the signs and symptoms of the disease. By looking outside of the box, it might provide a helpful treatment plan, which will give the patient a better quality of life.

Physicians and patients need to work together for the greater cause to help find relief and a cure for this misunderstood and complex disease we call CRPS.

Eric M. Phillips

INTRODUCTION

Eric M. Phillips

Complex regional pain syndrome (CRPS), formerly known as reflex sympathetic dystrophy (RSD) is a poorly understood syndrome by the medical community and the public. Many physicians are not familiar with the term CRPS, in turn, this lack of knowledge of the disease causes the patient to suffer for months to years without receiving a proper diagnosed or receive proper treatment.

CRPS is a painful disease which is caused by a minor injury, trauma, or surgery to an extremity. CRPS affects the patient physically, mentally, and emotionally. To obtain a complete understanding of this disease, physicians must conduct a careful history of the patient, learn, and understand the signs and symptoms of the disease.

As we are all well aware of CRPS is a complex disease to understand, diagnose, and to treat. CRPS is a multifaceted disease. CRPS affects each patient differently during the course of their disease. CRPS can affect men, woman, and children. It does not discriminate. The sad reality is CRPS can spread in some cases and it can also cause various complications such as, dysautonomia, immune system issues, loss of use

3

of the affected limb, spontaneous bruising and, urological issues in some patients. These are just a few of the various complications some patients may experience during the course of their disease.

CRPS affects millions of people worldwide. We must understand that CRPS is understood and treated differently around the world. There needs to be a global understanding on how CRPS develops, affects people, and how it should be treated.

CRPS affects individuals similarly, and it is essential to recognize that this condition is not in the patients head. Those affected all endure the same distressing experience of coping with constant, burning pain or an ice-cold pain sensation in the affected limb.

Unfortunately, many CRPS patients must fight daily to deal with their pain. At, times it is difficult for the patient to gain the proper help from the medical community, due to their lack of knowledge and understanding of the disease. There needs to be more recognition that CRPS is an actual disease.

With more education, research, and awareness, it will help us stop the pain that burns like an endless flame!

CHAPTER 1

THE DIFFERENCE BETWEEN COMPLEX REGIONAL PAIN SYNDROME (CRPS), FIBROMYALGIA(FM), AND MYOFASCIAL SYNDROME(MFS)

Eric M. Phillips

Abstract. Complex regional pain syndrome (CRPS) presents with a unique set of symptoms and pain that distinguishes it from any other syndrome or disorder recognized in modern medicine.

The symptoms of CRPS are often mistaken for other syndromes like fibromyalgia (FM) and myofascial syndrome (MFS). However, there is no comparison between CRPS and these syndromes. The pain and symptoms of CRPS are completely different from those of FM and MFS.

CRPS is a complex and painful syndrome to diagnosis and treat. The symptoms of CRPS can confuse the treating physician into thinking the patient may suffer from either FM, or MFS.

The lack of understanding about the complex pain of CRPS can lead to the delay in diagnosis and providing treatment for the patient.

5

There is a need for more education and awareness about the signs and symtoms of CRPS, so they are not confused with other syndrome such as FM or MFS.

Keywords. Complex regional pain syndrome (CRPS), fibromyalgia(FM), and myofascial syndrome (MFS).

INTRODUCTION

Over the course of several decades, there has been confusion between the symptoms of complex regional pain syndrome (CRPS) and other syndromes such as fibromyalgia (FM) and myofascial syndrome (MFS).

There is a big distinction between the signs and symptoms of CRPS, FM, and MFS. It is recognized that all these syndromes are painful in their own right, but the main symptoms are different. The one key symptom these painful syndromes share is the fatigue factor.

Unfortunately, many CRPS patients have been labeled as having both CRPS and FM. There are many differences between the two conditions. The medical community must realize that there is a major fatigue factor associated with CRPS. It should be noted that not every CRPS patient has FM (1).

In this chapter I will discuss more about the difference between CRPS, FM, and MFS.

THE HISTORY OF COMPLEX REGIONAL PAIN SYNDROME (CRPS)

In 1864, Doctor Silas Weir Mitchell the father of American neurology gave the description of causalgia in his classic article Gunshot Wounds and Other Injuries of Nerves, but it was not until 1867 when he coined the term of causalgia from the Greek words, "Kausos" (heat) and "algos" (pain) to describe this syndrome (2-4); in 1947, Doctor James Evans from Boston, named it Reflex Sympathetic Dystrophy Syndrome (RSDS), he also suggested doing a sympathetic nerve block, thinking that it might be useful for pain relief(2,5); in 1993; Doctor Hooshang Hooshmand described the four stages of RSD and the bilateral nature of RSD (2,6); and in 1994 Doctor Harold Merskey, et al, gave the disease the new official name of Complex Regional Pain Syndrome (CRPS) (2,7).

THE HISTORY OF FIBROMYALGIA

The symptoms of fibromyalgia(FM) have been documented for many centuries. In 1843, Doctor Robert Froriep from Germany, described symptoms of what we know today as FM(8). In 1904, the British neurologist Sir William Richard Gowers introduced the term fibrositis(9), while in 1972, Doctor Hugh Smythe coined the term fibromyalgia (10).

THE HISTORY OF MYOFASCIAL SYNDROME(MFS)

During the 16th century, Guillaume de Baillous, a French physician, was among the earliest to document muscle pain disorders(i.e., MFS)(11). In 1952, Doctors Janet Travell and Seymour Rinzler coined the term "myofascial trigger point(12)." Doctor Travell's, pioneer work on the subject of myofascial syndrome(MFS) has helped patients receive the proper diagnosis and treatment of this painful syndrome.

SIGNS AND SYMPTOMS OF CRPS

CRPS is a syndrome with multiple manifestations which require the following minimal symptoms and signs for the condition to be called CRPS (13).

- Pain: constant, burning pain, and in some forms at times during the course of the disease, stabbing type of pain (causalgic). The pain is relentless and is invariably accompanied by allodynia (even simple touch or breeze aggravating the pain) and hyperpathia (marked painful response to simple stimulation) (13).

8

- Spasms in the blood vessels of the skin and muscles of the extremities. The spasms in the blood vessels result in a very cold extremity. The muscle spasms result in a tremor, and movement disorders such as dystonia, flexion spasm, weakness, clumsiness of the extremities, and a tendency to fall(13).

- CRPS is accompanied by a certain degree of inflammation in practically all cases. This inflammation may be in the form of swelling (edema), skin rash (neurodermatitis), inflammatory changes of the skin color (mottled or purplish, bluish, or reddish or pale discolorations), a tendency for bleeding in the skin, skin becoming easily bruised, inflammation and swelling around the joints as well as in the joints (such as wrists, shoulders, knee, etc.) which can be identified on MRI in later stages, and secondary freezing of the joints(13).

- The fourth component and prerequisite of diagnosis of CRPS are insomnia, and emotional disturbance. The fact that the sympathetic sensory nerve fibers carrying the sympathetic pain and impulse up to the brain, terminate in the part of the brain

9

called "limbic system." This limbic (marginal) system which is positioned between the old brain (brainstem) and the new brain (cerebral hemispheres) is mainly located over the temporal and frontal lobes of the brain. The disturbance of function of these parts of the brain results in insomnia, agitation, depression, irritability, and disturbance of judgment. Insomnia is an integral part of an untreated CRPS case. So are problems of depression, irritability, and agitation(13).

So, the clinical diagnosis of CRPS is based on the above four principles rather than simply excluding CRPS and finding some other cause for the patient's pain(13).

According to Doctor Hooshmand, CRPS is not just the disease of peripheral nerves. The condition is not just a simple burning or stabbing pain. Besides the pain the patient also has other manifestations such as movement disorder, constriction of blood vessels in the extremity, swelling of the soft tissues (mistaken for "fibromyalgia"), and disturbance of the limbic system (the temporal-frontal lobe regions) (1,14).

Below are some of the symptoms associated with CRPS(13):

- Burning pain in the extremities.

- Chronic pain after injury or surgery.
- Cold feeling in the extremities.
- Discoloration of the skin.
- Edema (swelling of the extremities).
- Hypersensitivity to touch.
- Limited range of motion.
- Muscle spasms.

SIGNS AND SYMPTOMS OF FM

The specific cause of fibromyalgia(FM) is still unknown; however, studies suggest that individuals with this condition have an increased sensitivity to pain, which leads to their perception of pain when others may not feel it.

Below are some of the symptoms associated with FM:

- Body pain and stiffness(widespread pain).
- Fatigue.
- Depression and anxiety.
- Fatigue.
- Headaches (migraines).

11

- Memory and concentration issues.
- Sleep issues.
- Tiredness.

SIGNS AND SYMPTOMS OF MFS

The exact cause of myofascial syndrome (MFS) is still unknown. The symptoms of MFS can develop after a strain or injury to the muscles, ligaments, or tendons. Another cause is overuse of the muscle(i.e., repetitive movements).

Below are some of the symptoms associated with MFS:

- Fatigue.
- Headaches.
- Muscle stiffness.
- Poor sleep.
- Headaches.
- Postural abnormalities.
- Reduced range of motion.
- Sore and tender muscles.

- Weak muscles.

THE FATIGUE FACTOR IN CRPS

Understanding the distinctions between CRPS, FM, and MFS requires us to acknowledge that all three syndromes exhibit fatigue as a significant symptom.

The fatigue factor in CRPS coincides with the other symptoms found in CRPS(1).

The fatigue factor reported in CRPS patients has not been well documented in medical literature. The effects of living with the chronic pain of CRPS causes major fatigue. Not understanding the symptom of fatigue in CRPS, causes the patient to receive a misdiagnosis of either FM or MFS, which can cause a delay of receiving a proper diagnosis of CRPS for weeks, months, or years. This delay limits the patient from receiving proper treatment and pain relief(1).

THE DIFFERENCES BETWEEN CRPS AND FM

According to Doctor Littlejohn, the conditions of CRPS and FM can both be triggered by specific traumatic events, although FM is frequently associated with psychological trauma, and CRPS is commonly associated with physical trauma, which is often deemed routine or minor by the patient (1,15).

Lee and colleagues, reported that CRPS and FM share many features, both syndromes are chronic pain disorders which can cause severe pain, and both are considered to have a mechanism of action involving dysfunction of the sympathetic nervous system (SNS) (1,16).

The pain of CRPS, on the other hand, is more intense, being marked by burning, aching pain, fatigue, exhaustion, and a highly localized area of discomfort and pain. Compared to CRPS, FM causes less intense and widespread pain, as well as tenderness in the musculoskeletal system (1,16).

It should be noted that unlike FM, CRPS is usually accompanied by changes in skin color and skin temperature at the site of the original tissue injury, suggesting local sympathetic hyperactivity (1,15-17).

According to Doctor Hooshmand, CRPS patients are already at a disadvantage by being diagnosed as having FM, or MFS. This misdiagnosis can further delay the proper diagnosis and treatment (1,18).

The late Doctor Robert J. Schwartzman stated in his article Systemic Complications of CRPS published in 2012, that patients diagnosed with FM may also have CRPS. This is because the pressure points are part of the brachial plexus, the intercostobrachial (ICB) nerve, and the concomitant L5-S1 injury (19). He further states that the autonomic symptoms of CRPS are often mistaken for other disorders like fibromyalgia, Raynaud's phenomenon, and vascular insufficiency(19).

MYOFASCIAL SYNDROME (MFS) AND CRPS

Another syndrome a majority of CRPS patients are labeled with is myofascial syndrome (MFS). This is another misdiagnosis which can delay the patient from receiving a proper diagnosis and treatment for their pain(1).

According to Doctor Hooshmand, the term myofascial syndrome (MFS) refers to any soft tissue pain that cannot be specifically classified. It refers to a tender spot under the skin. That is all-nothing less nor nothing more. MFS is not accompanied by, "the cold, rapid hair growth, burning, and shooting pain, etc..." These are the symptoms of CRPS, but due to the nonspecific terminology of MFS, most CRPS patients are left untreated,

15

mistreated, and ignored until the disease becomes too advanced or too late to be managed (20).

CONCLUSION

Many CRPS patients have historically received misdiagnoses like fibromyalgia (FM) and myofascial syndrome (MFS) for decades. It is crucial to recognize the significant differences between CRPS and these other syndromes.

CRPS, FM, and MFS have been found to exhibit similar symptoms; however, the distinguishing feature of CRPS is the persistent burning or ice cold pain that patients endure. These particular symptoms are not observed in cases of FM or MFS. Recognizing the differences between these syndromes can greatly contribute to enhancing the quality of life for CRPS patients.

Further education and research is necessary to gain a comprehensive understanding of the differences between these painful syndromes, in order to facilitate an accurate diagnosis and effective treatment plan for patients.

16

A personal note: Unlike fibromyalgia, CRPS is a syndrome that is not widely recognized by the general public. My hope is that in the future, CRPS will receive the same level of recognition as fibromyalgia. Perhaps in the future, as we watch television, we might come across a commercial for a groundbreaking medication that effectively treats CRPS pain, and at that moment, everyone watching will be familiar with what CRPS stands for.

The initial documentation of CRPS in the United States dates back to 1864, during the American Civil War. However, it is imperative that we do not endure another 160 years for CRPS to receive widespread recognition among the general public.

REFERENCES

1. Phillips EM. The fatigue factor in complex regional pain syndrome (CRPS). In: Complex Regional Pain Syndrome (CRPS): Learning About The Different Aspects of a Painful Syndrome: Volume IV. Publisher: Amazon Books. 2023; Chapter 5: 69-78.

2. Phillips EM. The history of complex regional pain syndrome (CRPS). In: Complex Regional Pain Syndrome (CRPS): Learning About The Different Aspects of a Painful Syndrome: Volume I. Publisher: Amazon Books. 2022; Chapter 1: 5-18.

3. Hooshmand H, Phillips EM. Various complications of complex regional pain syndrome (CRPS). Feb 16, 2016. www.rsdinfo.com and www.rsdrx.com.

4. Mitchell SW, Morehouse GR, Keen WW. Gunshot Wounds and Other Injuries of Nerves. Philadelphia: Lippincott, 1864.

5. Evans JA. Reflex sympathetic dystrophy; report on 57 cases. Ann Intern Med 1947:26: 417-426.

6. Hooshmand H. Chronic Pain: Reflex Sympathetic Dystrophy: Prevention and Management. CRC Press, Boca Raton FL. 1993.

7. Merskey H, Bogduk N. Classification of chronic Pain Descriptions of Chronic Pain Syndromes and Definitions of Pain Terms. Task

Force on Taxonomy of the International Association for the Study of Pain. Merskey, H. editor. IASP Press. Seattle 1994.

8. Froriep R, On the Therapeutic Application of Electro-Magnetism in the Treatment of Rheumatic and Paralytic Affections, Translated by Lawrence RM, London, Henry Renshaw, 1850.

9. Gowers, W. R. A Lecture on lumbago: its lessons and analogues. Delivered at the National Hospital for the Paralysed and Epileptic. BMJ. 1904; 1, 117–121.

10. Smythe HA. Non-articular rheumatism and the fibrositis syndrome. Arthritis and allied conditions. 1972.

11. Guillaume de Baillou (1538–1616) clinician and epidemiologist. JAMA. 1966;195(11):957.

12. Travell JG, Rinzler SH. The myofascial genesis of pain. Postgrad Med. 1952; 11(5):425-434.

13. Phillips EM. Psychological aspect of complex regional pain syndrome (CRPS). In: Complex Regional Pain Syndrome (CRPS): Learning About The Different Aspects of a Painful Syndrome: Volume II. Publisher: Amazon Books. 2022; Chapter 10: 188-200.

14. Hooshmand H. RSD PUZZLE #32: "My RSD Started from An Injury To The Hand and After Carpal Tunnel Surgery. Why Is It I Can't Remember Anything?" 1997; www.rsdrx.com.

15. Littlejohn G. Neurogenic neuroinflammation in fibromyalgia and complex regional pain syndrome. Nat Rev Rheumatol 2015; 11:639.

16. Lee JY, Choi SH, Park KS, et al. Comparison of complex regional pain syndrome and fibromyalgia: Differences in beta and gamma bands on quantitative electroencephalography. Medicine (Baltimore). 2019 Feb;98(7): e14452.

17. Wurtman RJ. Fibromyalgia and the complex regional pain syndrome: similarities in pathophysiology and treatment. Metabolism 2010;59: S37–40.

20

18. Hooshmand H. RSD PUZZLE #121: Acupuncture in CRPS (RSD). 1997; www.rsdrx.com.

19. Schwartzman RJ. Systemic complications of complex regional pain syndrome. Neuroscience and Medicine 2012, 3, 225-242.

20. Hooshmand H. RSD PUZZLE #50: RSD By Any Other Name Is Still the Same. 1997; www.rsdrx.com.

CHAPTER 2

COMPLICATIONS CAUSED BY NERVE BLOCKS IN COMPLEX REGIONAL PAIN SYNDROME (CRPS) PATIENTS

Eric M. Phillips

Abstract. The first-line of treatment for complex regional pain syndrome (CRPS), is usually a series of sympathetic nerve block either a stellate ganglion block(SGB), or lumbar sympathetic nerve block(LSNB). These types of nerve blocks are performed as a diagnostic tool to back up a clinical diagnosis of CRPS, and as a therapeutic tool to help break the cycle of pain in the affected extremity.

The main purpose of performing these nerve blocks is to provide patients with relief from pain, which may last for a few hours, days, weeks, or even months.

In certain instances, patients may experience complications following a nerve block procedure. Some of these complications can be mild or more severe, which can create more pain or even spread of the patients symptoms.

The treating physician should properly inform the patient of the risks and complications that may arise from having any type of nerve block.

Keywords. Complex regional pain syndrome (CRPS), complications, lumbar sympathetic nerve block(LSNB), nerve blocks, sympathetic nerve block, stellate ganglion blocks (SGB).

INTRODUCTION

Nerve blocks have been utilized to help diagnose and alleviate the symptoms of complex regional pain syndrome (CRPS). There are many different types of nerve blocks used to treat CRPS. The main goal of performing a nerve block is to provide the patient with some form of pain relief. Unfortunately, some patients may not experience any pain relief and could potentially encounter complications as a result of the nerve block procedure. Some of these complications can be temporary or they can be permeant.

In this chapter I will discuss more about the complications caused by nerve blocks.

23

THE HISTORY OF NERVE BLOCKS

The use of nerve blocks with local anesthetics have been used for over a century. Doctor Carl Koller, an ophthalmologist from Vienna, Austria, discovered in 1884, that cocaine could be used for surgical local anesthesia. He conducted demonstrations to prove its effectiveness (1).

In 1885, Doctor James Leonard Corning, a New York neurologist, administered cocaine spinal anesthesia unintentionally. In his earlier research, he used hydrochlorate of cocaine, the only available local anesthetic at the time, first on the peripheral nervous system, then on the central nervous system. He noted that injecting cocaine under the skin caused both narrowing of blood vessels and numbing of the area.

Doctor Corning also conducted experiments using various types of injections, including interspinous and intentional intrathecal injections, to treat different neurological conditions (2,3).

Doctor August Karl Bier, a German physician, is known as the father of spinal and intravenous regional neural blockade. On August 16, 1898, he administered the first-ever spinal anesthesia using cocaine during a surgical procedure (4). He performed this procedure on six patients. All of them were successful in obtaining surgical anesthesia (4). In 1908,

Doctor Bier developed a new method of regional anesthesia known as intravenous regional anesthesia, also known as "Bier's-block(4,5)."

On December 30, 1899, Doctor Rudolph Matas from St. Charles Parish, Louisiana, is known for publishing the first account of spinal anesthesia in the United States. His account of spinal anesthesia during surgery was published in the Journal of the American Medical Association. A notable achievement of his, was the invention of the intravenous drip(6).

Doctor F. Dudley Tait, from San Francisco, California, and Doctor Guido E. Caglieri, from Italy, were the doctors who performed the first spinal anesthetic in the United States in 1900(7).

They performed a total of 11 spinal anesthetics. Three of them were cervical blocks and eight were lumbar blocks. Only six of 11 blocks performed resulted in adequate anesthesia, two blocks produced marginal results, and three were inadequate (7).

The pioneering work by Doctors Koller, Corning, Bier, Matas, Tait, and Caglieri has had a great impact on surgery, anesthesia, and treating CRPS worldwide.

STELLATE GANGLION BLOCKS (SGB) FOR CRPS

According to the late Doctor John J. Bonica who is considered the father of chronic pain management, as he specifies in his book, that the use of stellate ganglion blocks (SGB) in the best of hands (which would be Doctor Bonica) has a 25% rate of failure (8,9). This is because the stellate ganglion has a very vague anatomical structure which is different from patient to patient. So, it usually takes a few or several sticks before the ganglion block is done. A truly successful SGB is accompanied by Horner's syndrome (oculosympathetic paralysis) (8,10,11).

It is unfortunate that some people continue to undergo SGB despite the fact that it has caused complete destruction of the sympathetic ganglion nerve cell, and the patient has experienced a traumatic sympathectomy, as evidenced by a warm and dry hand and forearm (8).

When the ganglion cannot be reached because of anatomical variations, then the repeated trauma while performing the block can cause damage to the nerve in the vocal cord causing difficulty with phonation (speaking). It also can cause rupture of blood vessels in the same area(8).

A SGB is mainly a traumatic diagnostic procedure, it cannot be considered therapeutic because it does not last more than a few hours to a few days.

26

When performing an epidural block, you do not stick the needle into the nerve cells (as is the case with SGB). When an epidural block is performed, with local anesthetic and an anti-inflammatory medication such as Depo-Medrol ® in the back of the neck, it will last from two to three months(8).

COMPLICATIONS CAUSED BY STELLATE GANGLION BLOCKS (SGB)

Stellate ganglion blocks(SGB) are the standard nerve blocks for neuropathic pain such as CRPS. However, these blocks are not consistently successful and they can cause some complications (8,9,12-16).

SGB can be performed by using the following three approaches:

- Using the traditional landmark-based approach.
- Using the image guidance of fluoroscopy.
- Using the image guidance of ultrasound.

According to Goel, et al., complications of SGB can be divided into two groups; systemic and local(17).

- Systemic complications: this form of complication is a result of the medication entering into an unintended space or it can cause the body to have an allergic reaction(17).

- Local complications: this form of complication is due to unintentional injury to the structure in the path of the needle(17).

The following is a list of systemic complications and local complications of SGB (17).

Systemic complications:

- Allergic reaction.
- Bilateral Horner's Syndrome.
- Contralateral Horner's Syndrome.
- Cough.
- Headache(Migraine)
- Hoarseness.
- Hypertension.
- Light-headiness.
- Numbness of the arm.
- Seizures.

- Respiratory Depression.

Local complications:

- Asystolic cardiac arrest.
- Blood aspiration.
- Bradycardia.
- Dural puncture.
- Hematoma.
- Infection.
- Pneumothorax.
- Sinus arrest.

In 2022, Goel and colleagues, performed a systematic review on complications associated with SGNB. They reviewed published complications caused by SGB, which were reported between 1990-2018. In their research they found 67 medical articles reporting complications from SGNB, with a total of 260 cases that had developed complications from undergoing SGB (17).

They also noted that complications have been reported in connection with the landmark-based technique, as well as with the use of fluoroscopy and ultrasound guidance. The SGB were performed for different types of chronic pain conditions such as CRPS, postherpetic neuralgia, brachial plexus injury, and postoperative pain control(17).

Out of the 260 cases of complications related to SGB, 36 (13.8%) occurred in women, 24 (9.2%) occurred in men, and the remaining 200 (76.9%) cases were unspecified because they were part of a larger series(17).

The use of image guidance was utilized for SGB in 134 of the 260 (51.5%) cases. They reported that 64 patients (24.6%) had undergone SGB with use of ultrasound and 70 patients (26.9%) had undergone SGB with use fluoroscopy guidance. Complications were observed when using both of these forms of guidance. The use of landmark-only guidance was performed on 126 patients (48.5%)(17).

In their research, they found a total of 172 patients (68.4%) who experienced medication-related or systemic side effects, and 82 patients (31.5%) experienced procedure-related or local side effects. Unfortunately, one person passed away because of a massive hematoma that caused airway obstruction(17).

In 2004, Saxena, et al., reported on a case of a 29-year-old female patient who suffered from chronic right shoulder-hand pain. She underwent a right-side SGB. During the procedure the patient developed a sinus arrest, she also had apnea, unconsciousness, and persistent postural hypotension, which lasted for 24-hours. Her symptoms from the complications from the SGB lasted 10-minutes(18).

Kimura, et al., reported in 2005, that seven patients who had undergone SGB all developed complications of severe hypertension (19).

In 2005, Balaban and colleagues, reported on a case of a 21-year-old male with CRPS who underwent a SGB on the right-side, using the landmark-based approach. The patient had previously undergone 11 SGB without any issues. Twenty-five minutes after the patient underwent his 12th SGB, he had developed severe stridor(high-pitched respiratory sound caused by a narrowed airway),apnea, and paralysis of all four extremities. These symptoms lasted for three hours after the procedure(20).

In a 2009, case study by Eyigor and colleagues, documented a case involving a 16-year-old girl diagnosed with CRPS. The patient received a SGB on the right side under fluoroscopy guidance. However, the administration of a 5 mg dose of Lidocaine during the procedure led to the occurrence of grand mal seizures, loss of consciousness, and respiratory arrest(21).

Atici and Akoz, reported in 2010, a CRPS patient developed a transient cough after her forth SGB. The cough only lasted one to two hours after the procedure(22).

Doctors Sari and Aydin reported in 2012, on a case of a 44-year-old female who was undergoing a SGB for the diagnosis of CRPS. Unfortunately, this patient developed respiratory arrest, four to five minutes after the SGB was performed(23).

In 2013, Doctor C.H. Kim, reported a case of a 43-year-old woman with CRPS who underwent a right-side SGB under fluoroscopy guidance. The procedure was performed with a low dose of 3 ml of 0.25% bupivacaine. The SGB caused the patient to develop complications related to respiratory depression. During the procedure the patient complained she was having difficulties breathing. For several hours, she required intubation and ventilation support(24).

In 2017, Datta, et al., reported that out of 287 nerve block injections, there were 33 complications with a total rate of 11.1%. The complications were all minor and self-limiting(25).

HORNER'S SYNDROME(HS) COMPLICATIONS IN CRPS

A Horner's syndrome(HS) is successfully achieved in around 75% of the patients who undergo SGB. It also has other serious complications which would be harmful to the patients (8,10,11).

The below are the complications of HS in CRPS patients:

- Anhidrosis (decreased sweating).
- Enopthalmos (eyeball sinking into face).
- Flushed reddish appearance of the face
- Headaches.
- Hoarseness of the voice.
- Miosis (constricted pupil).
- Ptosis (drooping eyelid).
- The eyes may show a different color.

According to Datta, et al., they reported symptoms of HS develop after SGB, which is evidence of a successful SGB. However, the sign of HS, does not always confirm a complete and successful SGB(25).

VIRTUAL SYMPATHECTOMY COMPLICATION IN CRPS

Virtual sympathectomy is another complication caused by repetitive nerve blocks, seen in some cases of CRPS.

The term of virtual sympathectomy was coined in 1998, by my mentor the late Doctor Hooshang Hooshmand (8,26). Doctor Hooshmand reported that doing both repetitive stellate ganglion blocks (SGB) or a repetitive lumbar sympathetic nerve blocks(LSNB) can cause a virtual sympathectomy (Figures. 1 and 2) (8,26).

The worst feature of the SGB is the fact that repeated SGB result in the bombardment and traumatic needle damage to the stellate ganglion sympathetic nerve cells. God created those nerve cells not to be needled and destroyed. Quite frequently, after several SGB, the patient develops sympathetically independent pain (SIP) in a patient who before the ganglion blocks had sympathetically maintained pain (SMP) (8).

This confuses the clinician and because a successful block does not help the patient anymore, and the patient is accused of being a malingerer or not having "CRPS anymore". Frequently, in such patients the hand and forearm or the foot and leg become warm and stay warm because of the

34

virtual sympathectomy due to the needling of the stellate ganglion (Figure. 1) (8,14,26-28).

Infrared thermal imaging (ITI) is a very useful tool which helps identify the damage from the virtual sympathectomy which is caused by repetitive SGB and LSNB (8,14,26-28).

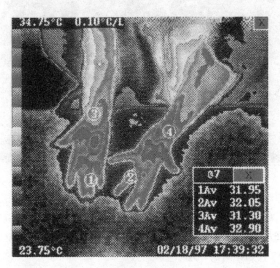

Figure 1. More than two dozen stellate ganglion blocks(SGB) to each side have damaged enough sympathetic nerve to cause permanent

35

hyperthermia as the manifestation of virtual sympathectomy. Further blocks have no diagnostic or therapeutic value. With the use of infrared thermal imaging (ITI), it spared the patient from further sympathetic nerve blocks (8,14).

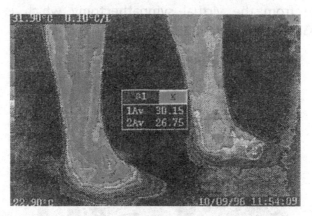

Figure 2. "Virtual sympathectomy" due to repetitive right lumber sympathetic nerve blocks, resulting in permanent damage and heat leakage in lower extremity. The patient was spared from further nerve blocks on the right side (8,26).

CONCLUSION

The use of SGB to treat CRPS and other pain conditions can cause many different types of complications which have been documented over the past few decades. These complications can be mild to severe, and they can be temporary or permanent.

The hopes of performing a SGB or LSNB is to provide the patient with some form of pain relief and a better quality of life.

Complications associated with SGB have been reported using three different approaches such as the landmark-based approach, fluoroscopy guidance, and ultrasound guidance.

There are two group types associated with SGB complications: systemic complications(i.e., allergic reaction, bilateral Horner's syndrome, contralateral Horner's syndrome, and cough) and local complications (i.e., Asystolic cardiac arrest, blood aspiration, bradycardia, hematoma).

Another complication seen in CRPS patients, which has been reported and documented by Doctor Hooshmand, is the damage caused by repetitive sympathetic blocks, which causes a "virtual sympathectomy"(8,14,26-28). Virtual sympathectomy is caused by the

37

repeated repetitive sympathetic blocks, which results in the bombardment and traumatic needle damage to the stellate ganglion sympathetic nerve cells (8).

Performing repetitive sympathetic blocks, which result in virtual sympathectomy, can lead to the spread of CRPS and exacerbate the patient's pain.

It is essential for the treating physician to inform the patient about the potential risks and complications that can arise from SGB and other types of nerve blocks.

REFERENCES

1. Koller C. The use of cocaine for producing anaesthesia on the eye. Lancet. 1884;2:990.

2. Corning JL. A further contribution on local medication of the spinal cord, with cases. Medical Record. 1888; 17;33(11):291.

3. Corning JL. Pain. Philadelphia: JB Lippincott. 1894.

4. Bier A. Uber einen neuen Weg Lokalanasthsie und den GliedmaBen zu erzeugen. Arch. Klin. Chir. 1908;86:1007-1016.

5. Bier A. Ueber Venenanasthesie. (On venous anesthesia) Berliner Klinische Wochenschrift. 1909; 46:477-489.

6. Matas R. Local and regional anesthesia: A retrospect and prospect. Am J Surg. 1934; 189–196 and August 1934; 362–379.

7. Tait D, Caglieri G. Experimental and clinical notes on the subarachnoid space, JAMA. 1900; 35: 6-10.

8. Phillips EM. Complex Regional Pain Syndrome (CRPS): Learning About The Different Aspects Of A Painful Syndrome: Volume III. Amazon Books. 2023. Chapter 11; 164-179.

9. Bonica JJ: The Management of Pain. Lea & Feibger Philadelphia. 1990; Vol. 1: p 229.

10. Elias M. Cervical Sympathetic and Stellate Ganglion Blocks. Pain Physician. 2000; 3: 294-304.

11. Amhaz HH, Manders L. Chidiac EJ, et al. Unusual case of contralateral Horner's syndrome following stellate-ganglion block: a case report and review of the literature. Local Reg Anesth. 2013; 6: 31–33.

12. Hooshmand, H., Hashmi, M., Phillips, EM. Nerve Blocks for Neuropathic Pain. Abstracts of the 10th World Congress on Pain. San Diego, California, August 19, 2002. International Association for the Study of Pain (IASP Press) Page 208, Number 638- P272.

13. Carr DB, Cepeda MS, Lau J. What is the evidence for the therapeutic role of local anesthetic sympathetic blockade in RSD or causalgia? An attempted meta-analysis [abstract] Eighth world congress on pain, Vancouver, August 17-22 1996., Seattle: IASP Press. 1996; 406.

14. Hooshmand H, Hashmi H. Complex regional pain syndrome (CRPS, RSDS) diagnosis and therapy. A review of 824 patients. Pain Digest. 1999; 9: 1-24.

15. Kozin F. Reflex sympathetic dystrophy: a review. Clin Exp Rheumatol. 1992; 10: 401-409.

16. Schott GD. Interrupting the sympathetic outflow in causalgia and reflex sympathetic dystrophy. A futile procedure for many patients. BMJ. 1998; 316: 792-793.

17. Goel V, Patwardhan AM, Ibrahim M, et al. Complications associated with stellate ganglion nerve block: a systematic review. Reg Anesth Pain Med. 2019; 1-23.

18. Saxena AK, Saxena N, Aggarwal B, et al. An unusual complication of sinus arrest following right-sided stellate ganglion block: a case report. Pain Pract. 2004; 4:245-248.

19. Kimura T, Nishiwaki K, Yokota S, et al. Severe hypertension after stellate ganglion block. British Journal of Anaesthesia. 2005; 94: 840-842.

20. Balaban B, Baklaci K, Taskaynatan MA, et al. Delayed subdural block as an unusual complication following stellate ganglion blockade. The Pain Clinic. 2005;17:407–409.

21. Eyigor C, Erhan E, Yegul I. Grand mal seizure following stellate ganglion block after negative aspiration. Pain Practice. 2009; 9: 37–38.

22. Atici S, Akoz K. Transient cough attacks after right stellate ganglion block. Reg Anesth Pain Med. 2010; 35: 318-319.

23. Sari S, Aydin ON. Intraspinal blockade after stellate ganglion blockade in trauma patient. Reg Anesth Pain Med. 2012;37:E239–E240.

24. Kim CH. Respiratory depression following stellate ganglion block. PM&R. 2013;5.

25. Datta R, Agrawal J, Sharma A, et al. A study of the efficacy of stellate ganglion blocks in complex regional pain syndromes of the upper body. J Anaesthesiol Clin Pharmacol. 2017; 33: 534–540.

26. Hooshmand H. Is thermal imaging of any use in pain management? Pain Digest. 1998; 8:166-170.

27. Hooshmand, H., Hashmi, M, Phillips, EM. Infrared thermal imaging as a tool in pain management. An 11-year study, Part I of II, Thermology International. 2001; 11: 53-65.

28. Hooshmand H, Hashmi M, Phillips, EM. Infrared thermal imaging as a tool in pain management. An 11- year study, Part II: Clinical Applications. Thermology International. 2001; 11: 1-13.

43

CHAPTER 3

TREATMENT WITH ICE CAN CAUSE COMPLICATIONS IN COMPLEX REGIONAL PAIN SYNDROME (CRPS)

Eric M. Phillips

Abstract. Complex regional pain syndrome (CRPS) is a painful syndrome with the main symptom being unrelenting burning pain. The effects of CRPS can make the patient feel like their affected limb is on fire 24/7, which is one of the most painful situations any human can ever endure. To alleviate this unbearable feeling of the "fire from hell," most patients would opt to apply ice to their painful burning limb to help reduce the feeling of unrelenting burning pain.

Unfortunately, the application of ice to treat the painful symptoms of CRPS, can cause more pain, spread of the disease, and can cause permanent damage to myelinated nerves.

The treating physician, physical therapist, and occupational therapist should be aware of the dangers of applying ice to an affected CRPS extremity.

It is important that patients should avoid this form of treatment to prevent creating more pain and the potential of causing their CRPS to spread.

Keywords. Complex regional pain syndrome (CRPS), application of ice, cryosurgery, cryoablation, skin necrosis, and spread of CRPS.

INTRODUCTION

According to my mentor the late Doctor Hooshmand, the application of ice is the treatment of choice for acute soft tissue injuries, and it is contraindicated in the treatment of CRPS. Ice is also an instigator, aggravator, and perpetuator of CRPS due to its vasoconstrictive effect(1).

The use of cryotherapy (the application of ice) can cause permanent somatosensory and thermosensory (sympathetic) nerve damage (2).

Repetitive application of ice may result in further sympathetic nerve dysfunction causing blotching of the skin(2).

The application of cryosurgery (cryoablation) with the application of liquid nitrogen is fraught with a higher risk of causing nerve damage (2,3).

It is important for all CRPS patients to be cautious of the impact of using ice on their affected limb. If they experience heightened pain or worsening symptoms, they must discontinue ice application promptly to avoid exacerbating the condition.

In this chapter I will discuss more about the damage the application of ice can cause to a CRPS patient.

COMPLICATIONS CAUSED BY ICE IN CRPS

In 2004, Doctor Hooshmand and I had published a case study of a CRPS patient who had developed CRPS in her right knee in June 1996, from a sports related injury(2). It took two years for the patient to receive an official diagnosis of CRPS.

At the scene of the accident, the application of ice was applied. For a span of almost five years the patient applied ice to her knee two to three times a day(2).

Prior to the patients referral to Doctor Hooshmand's clinic in May of 2001, she had already undergone the following procedures(2):

- Arthroscopy of the right knee.
- Multiple sympathetic ganglion nerve blocks (which had failed).
- Twelve Bier blocks (which caused further exacerbation of signs and symptoms).

46

- Cryotherapy, and cryosurgery of the right saphenous nerve and vein.

The cryotherapy, and cryosurgery she had undergone, led to neuroinflammation in the form of edema, bulbous lesions, and multiple trophic ulcers over the right knee, hyperthermia, and intractable pain (Figure 1) (2).

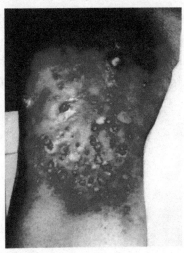

Figure 1. Five years of daily self-applied cryotherapy(ice application)resulted in the breakdown of skin, cold blisters, and damage to sensory nerves (2).

47

In March of 1999, the patient began to experience multiple skin ulcers on her right knee. By November of 2000, she had counted more than 250 ulcers on the right knee(2).

When she was first seen at Doctor Hooshmand's clinic, the application of ice was discontinued. During her evaluation, she was found to have marked edema above and below the right knee (Figure 1) (2).

She underwent infrared thermal imaging (ITI), which showed marked hypothermia on the right patellar region 15 cm in height and 12 cm in width, with a temperature of 22.75° C. This was in contrast to the left knee temperature which was 28° C (DT = 5.25° C), confirming severe vasoconstriction due to CRPS (Figure 2) (2).

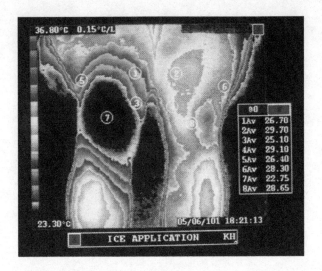

Figure 2. Bilateral thermogram shows marked hypothermia due to vasoconstriction in the cryotherapy area(2).

The patient underwent the standard treatment protocol for neuropathic pain (2). Her edema and bulbous lesions were treated with intravenous mannitol resulting in resolution of the lesions (Figure 3) (2,4,5).

49

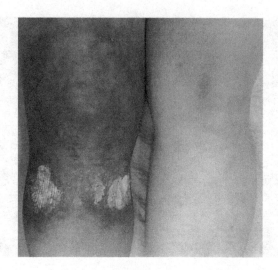

Figure 3. Eleven days after discontinuation of cryotherapy, treatment of epidural, regional nerve blocks, and intravenous mannitol, showed marked improvement of the bulbous lesions(2).

The treatment she had undergone included, the following medications and procedures (2):

Medications:

- Analgesic antidepressant treatment with (trazodone and venlafaxine).

50

- Discontinuation of cryotherapy.
- Emla and doxepin cream (alternated).
- Epsom salt (magnesium sulfate) soaks.
- Intravenous mannitol(to reduce the neuroinflammation)
- Stadol (butorphanol) nasal spray.
- Tramadol

Procedures:

- Femoral nerve blocks containing bupivacaine and Depo-Medrol®.
- Lumbar epidural nerve blocks containing Depo-Medrol®.

The nerve blocks she underwent provided marked improvement in circulation in the lower extremities (2).

After 11 days of treatment, the patient's knee warmed up for the first time since 1996. Her blisters and bullae on her knee had cleared. She rated her pain at a two (on the basis of 0-10) (Figure 3) (2).

51

With the help of taking trazodone, it suppressed the nocturnal pain, and for the first time in five years, she was able to sleep eight hours a night without interruption(2).

In addition, the epidural and femoral blocks helped reduce the right knee hypothermia which reversed it to hyperthermia (Figure 3). The nerve blocks dilated the arterioles resulting in further hyperthermia and improved tissue oxygenation(2).

In 2008, Nishikawa, et al., reported a case of a 36-year-old woman with CRPS, who developed extensive skin necrosis of the left arm. The patient used ice packs to cool her arm to alleviate the severe burning pain she was experiencing from the symptoms of CRPS. She was informed that if she uses ice repeatedly, it could lead to a frostbite injury. The area of skin necrosis correlates with the area where she had applied ice packs to cool her affected limb (6).

ICE AND HEAT TOLERANCE IN CRPS

For decades, there has been an ongoing discussion regarding the effectiveness of ice and heat treatment in managing the symptoms of CRPS.

It is vital that the treating physician, physical therapist, and occupational therapist understand how CRPS patients tolerate the application of ice and heat. Also, they must understand the damage that ice can cause to an affected CRPS extremity.

In the 1990's, Doctor Hooshmand performed a study on ice tolerance versus heat tolerance among CRPS. In his study he found that 87% of the patients could not tolerate cold, and 13% could not tolerate heat(7).

In his study he utilized infrared thermal imaging(ITI) which showed the patients who could not tolerate heat (13%) had advanced stages of sympathetic nerve paralysis rather than nerve irritation (death of the sympathetic nerve fibers rather than hyperactive nerve fibers). The area of permanent sympathetic nerve damage in late stage of the disease acted like a leaky radiator, causing leakage of heat through the skin which resulted in warm extremity and secondary intolerance to external heat, meaning that due to permanent damage to the sympathetic nerve fibers (after repeated ganglion nerve blocks or sympathectomy) the sympathetic nerves could not contain and preserve the heat originating from the deep structures of muscle, bone, etc... (7).

He mentioned in his study that a small portion (13%) of patients did not exhibit the hyperactive cold vasoconstriction of the skin, which is typically seen in the early stages of CRPS. These patients, who are

53

intolerant to heat, would be categorized as having erythromelalgia. In contrast, the remaining 87% of CRPS patients experience hyperactive sympathetic function, resulting in cold extremities and intolerance to cold exposure. However, if ice is applied repeatedly, it can freeze and coagulate the myelin, which is similar to what happens when ice freezes and solidifies melted butter. When the ice freezes and damages the myelinated nerves, the patient experiences sensory loss and pain because the large nerve fibers are permanently damaged(7).

The addition of sensory nerve pain, which is not originating from sympathetic sources exacerbates the CRPS alongside the initial thermal sensory pain(7).

The use of ice leads to complete anesthesia and pain relief for a few minutes, similar to the numbness experienced when the hand comes into contact with a snowball in the winter time(7).

HOT AND COLD CHALLENGE TREATMENT IN CRPS

According to Doctor Hooshmand, the application of hot and cold challenge in the management of CRPS during physical therapy or occupational therapy can be harmful and cause exacerbation of the patients pain(8).

In addition, Doctor Hooshmand mentions when the skin is cold and blue, it is a sign of vasoconstriction. In the early stages of the disease, exposure to cold, whether through ice or cold water, exacerbates the vasoconstriction(8).

In contrast, when the extremity is warm, it indicates damage to the thermoreceptors. This causes heat to leak from deeper structures. Patients who experience this usually have a low tolerance for heat. The reason for this is damage to vasoconstrictors, which allows heat to enter the body and the condition becomes worse(8).

Applying ice and hot water to the injured area worsens the condition by causing neurovascular instability, resulting in blotching and unstable thermoregulation(8).

To prevent damage to the affected area, Doctor Hooshmand advises against applying hot and cold challenge treatments to the affected area in the management of CRPS.

THE RED FLAGS OF USING ICE IN CRPS TREATMENT

CRPS patients and their treating medical team should be aware of the red flags that are associated with the application of ice for the treatment of CRPS.

The red flag warning signs of ice application should be discontinued if the patient develops any of the following symptoms:

- Blotching of the skin.
- Bulbous lesions.
- Hyperthermia.
- Intractable pain.
- Spread of CRPS symptoms.
- Trophic ulcers.

CONCLUSION

The application of ice is useful for treatment of acute pain. However, prolonged, and repetitive application of ice can cause permanent nerve damage(2).

56

According to Doctor Hooshmand, the application of ice results in stimulation of the sympathetic system and secondary constriction of the superficial sympathetic vasoconstrictors(9).

I have personally suffered from CRPS for over 38-years and I totally understand what every CRPS patient deals with daily. I understand the unrelenting burning pain that is associated with CRPS, and I understand the thought process of patients dealing with a limb on fire, and wanting to put out the fire that never goes away.

The first line of thinking for each and every CRPS patient and their medical team is to apply ice to the affected limb or stick it into a bucket of cold water. This theory would work if someone was putting out a real fire, but when it comes to the burning pain of CRPS it is a different story. The application of ice can cause permanent damage to myelinated nerves, which can also cause the patient to have more pain and spread of the disease.

It is vital to understand the dangers of the application of ice in the management of CRPS. Patients and their treating medical team must work together on other treatment plans, other than applying ice to an already painful limb. Applying ice in the treatment of CRPS should be avoided at all cost. Ice and CRPS do not mix, and it is a recipe for disaster and more pain for the patient.

REFERENCES

1. Hooshmand H. Chronic Pain: Reflex Sympathetic Dystrophy: Prevention and Management. CRC Press, Boca Raton FL. Textbook; 1993.

2. Hooshmand H, Hashmi M, Phillips EM. Cryotherapy can cause permanent nerve damage: A case report. American Journal of Pain Management. 2004; 14: 2: 63-70.

3. Wingfield DL, Fraunfelder FT. Possible complications secondary to cryotherapy. Opthalmic Surg 1979; 10:47-55.

4. Hooshmand H, Dove J, Houff S , et al. Effects of diuretics and steroids in CSF pressure, a comparative study. Arch Neurol. 1969; 21:499-509.

5. Veldman PH, Goris RJ. Sequelae of reflex sympathetic dystrophy. In: Clinical Aspects of Reflex Sympathetic Dystrophy. Koninklijke Biblioteek, Den Haag, Netherlands: 1995:119-129.

6. Nishikawa M, Tanioka M, Araki E, et al. Extensive skin necrosis of the arm in a patient with complex regional pain syndrome. Clin Exp Dermatol. 2008; 33(6):733-735.

7. Hooshmand H. RSD Puzzle #102. Ice versus Heat. 1997. www.rsdrx.com

8. Hooshmand H. RSD Puzzle #145. Hot and Cold Challenge in the Treatment of Early Stages of RSD/CRPS. 1997. www.rsdrx.com

9. Hooshmand H. RSD Puzzle #5. Why Not Use Ice for RSD Therapy? 1996. www.rsdrx.com

CHAPTER 4

MULTIPLE LIMB AND TOTAL BODY
COMPLEX REGIONAL PAIN SYNDROME (CRPS)

Eric M. Phillips

Abstract. Complex regional pain syndrome (CRPS) is an extremely painful and complex syndrome to diagnose and treat.

CRPS has been documented throughout history to affect both the upper and lower extremities for centuries, with instances of patients experiencing CRPS in multiple limbs(ML-CRPS) and even developing total-body CRPS(TB-CRPS).

The spread of CRPS into multiple limbs or total body is a serious problem for many patients during the course of their disease. Most physicians treating CRPS patients do not understand or believe that CRPS can spread. They feel that CRPS is a one-dimensional syndrome and it cannot spread. It can be frustrating when healthcare providers dismiss symptoms of spread as being "all in the patient's head."

Unfortunately, the sad reality is CRPS can spread into other limbs and also cause total body symptoms. However, it should be emphasized that not every patient with CRPS will develop it in multiple limbs or experience the total-body spread of the disease.

It is vital for all physicians who treat CRPS patients should not overlook or dismiss the fact CRPS can spread to other parts of the body or into the internal organs (1-3).

The key to prevent any form of spread of CRPS is with treatments of nerve blocks, medications, physical and occupational therapy. This is a starting point to prevent spread of the disease.

Keywords. Bilateral spread, complex regional pain syndrome (CRPS), multiple limb-CRPS(ML-CRPS), reflex sympathetic dystrophy (RSD), single limb-CRPS (SL-CRPS), spread of CRPS, and total body-CRPS (TB-CRPS).

INTRODUCTION

The spread of CRPS can develop in any of the first three stages of the disease (1,3-8). Some cases of spread can happen within weeks to months after the initial onset of the disease or some cases can take years to develop spread into multiple limbs or total body involvement.

61

According to the late Doctor Robert J. Schwartzman, CRPS is a progressive illness which can spread over time and may encompass the entire body. Despite the absence of a psychological disposition, all patients suffer from severe depression as a result of the persistent pain, sleep deprivation, and complete disruption of their lifestyle (9).

In my time working with my mentor the late Doctor Hooshmand, we had seen cases of spread early in the course of the disease and cases which took years to decades to spread. As, I have always said, CRPS has a mind of its own and it will do what it wants, when it wants to do it. Some patients are very fortunate not to develop spread of the disease at all.

In the late stages of CRPS, due to prolonged immobilization, or improper treatment such as unnecessary surgery or application of ice, the disease shows a tendency to spread (1,11). The spread of CRPS may be vertical from arm to leg (or vice versa) on the same side or may be horizontal from arm to arm or leg to leg. The spread which occurs in about one third of patients is more likely to develop after surgical procedure (1,8,10-19).

The phenomenon of spread (either multiple limbs or total body) in CRPS patients have been reported by Doctors Hooshmand, Schwartzman, Veldman, Maleki, Kozin, Radt, and many others (1,4-7,20).

In this chapter, I will discuss how CRPS can spread. The spread of CRPS can be caused by many factors, such as surgery, another injury or on its own (1).

SPREAD OF CRPS

In 1939, Doctor René Leriche and in 1945, Doctor Geza de Takats observed that patients with CRPS may encounter burning pain solely in the initial area. However, in certain instances, the condition can extend to other body parts, and in rare cases, it can affect the entire body(21,22).

The spread of CRPS is not usually limited to one part of an extremity or one extremity. Usually, the pathological sympathetic function spreads to adjacent areas (1,11). CRPS can also spread to the orofacial region; it causes necrosis (death of cells) of the maxillary and mandibular bones in the areas of the root canals. It can also spread internally in some cases (1,8).

The mechanism of spread is due to the fact that at the level of the spinal cord, the sympathetic input has a tendency to cross the midline to the opposite side. The second reason for spread is a chain of relay stations of the sympathetic nerves in the form of sympathetic ganglia on each side of the spine (1,8,18).

In Doctor Hooshang Hooshmand's textbook on reflex sympathetic dystrophy (RSD), he reported the chain of sympathetic ganglia from the base of the skull to sacral regions on the right and left sides, typically spread the pathologic impulse to other extremities (1,4).

The research by Kozin, et al., shows that CRPS can spread vertically or horizontally in both upper or both lower extremities (1,3,5). Also, undergoing any surgical procedure can promote the potential spread of CRPS (1-3,7). Maleki, et al., published a retrospective analysis of 27 CRPS patients. In this study, all 27 patients had experienced a spread of their pain (1,3,20).

In a 2002, study by Doctor Fiona Greatorex, reported it has been observed that CRPS can cause both pain and abnormal sensations to spread from the initial area to other parts of the body. This suggests that a central component may play a significant role in contributing to the syndrome's symptoms(23).

BILATERAL SPREAD OF CRPS

In 1943, Doctor William K. Livingston coined the term "mirror images". He had reported "mirror images" in 35 patients with bilateral symptoms of CRPS(17).

The main reason for the CRPS becoming bilateral and spreading to other extremities is because in contrast to the somatic nervous system, the sympathetic nervous system has bilateral innervation. In the somatic nervous system (usual sensation and motor function) the abnormalities in dermatome in a specific nerve root distribution, whereas in CRPS the abnormality is distributed among the blood vessels, distribution of nerves (Thermatomes) and to the sympathetic ganglia and then across the midline collections, the condition reflects itself on both sides rather than one side of the body. This bilateral manifestation through the sympathetic plexi across the midline explains the patient's problem with headache, dizziness, tinnitus, chest pain, and abdominal manifestations of CRPS (gastritis, diarrhea, cramps) and spread of CRPS to other extremities (1,8).

MULTIPLE LIMB CRPS(ML-CRPS)

In 1996, Doctors Veldmand and Goris from the Netherlands reviewed 1183 CRPS cases, between 1984-1994(5).

They reviewed two groups, consisting of patients with single limb-CRPS (SL-CRPS) and patients with multiple limb-CRPS(ML-CRPS)(5).

The group with single-limb CRPS comprised of 1,065 patients (5):

- 798 females(75%).
- 267 males(20%).

The group with multiple limb-CRPS comprised of 118 patients(5):

- 95 females(80%).
- 23 males(20%).

The first location of CRPS was reported in the upper extremity in 58 patients (49%) and 60 patients (51%) with lower limb involvement(5).

In their study they found no difference between patients who only had CRPS in one limb versus patients who had CRPS in multiple limbs(5).

In 2000, Doctor Maleki and colleagues, identified three distinct patterns of spread observed in patients with CRPS(20).

Below are the three distinct patterns of spread seen in CRPS patients(20):

- Contiguous spread: which is characterized by gradual enlargement of the area affected from the distal to more proximal regions of the limb(20).

- Independent spread: which is seen in 70% of patients, depicted by the appearance of signs and symptoms at the site distant and noncontagious from the initial site of CRPS(20

- Mirror-image spread: this type of spread is seen in 15% of patients typified by the appearance of symptoms in the opposite limb in a region similar to the original injury site(20).

In 2007, Doctors Khand and Scarlet, reviewed a case of a 45-year-old male who developed CRPS in all four limbs after having an electric shock in his righthand. The injury occurred while the patient was working with an electrical generator. He received an electric shock of 6000 volts when he touched a power source. He had an entry wound in the right palm, and an exit wound in his right foot(24).

The patient was in the hospital for 12 days. Three to four months after the electric shock injury, the patient started to develop pain in the right upper and lower limbs and burning sensation in all the four limbs. The patient met all the necessary diagnostic criteria for CRPS and was formally diagnosed (24).

67

In 2011, Doctor van Rijn, et at., reviewed 185 CRPS patients. Ninety-six patients(52%) had SL-CRPS. Eighty-nine patients(48%) had ML-CRPS. They also reported that 78 patients had developed spread into another limb(25).

They observed, that the severity of CRPS symptoms in the second limb was comparable to the first limb, with no significant variation (25).

They reported three different patterns of spread among 72 patients in their study(25).

- Contralateral pattern: 38 patients (53%) (22 arm to arm, and 16 leg to leg).

- Ipsilateral pattern: 23 patients (32%) (12 arm to leg, and 11 leg to arm).

- Diagonal pattern: 11 patients (15%).

They also reported that a new trauma caused spread of CRPS into a second limb in(25):

- 37% of the patients with contralateral spread.

- 44% of the patients with ipsilateral spread.

- 91% of the patients with diagonal spread(which is always associated with a new trauma).

Spread after a separate trauma was reported in 34 patients who had trauma to a second limb(25).

- Contralateral spread: 14 patients (41%) (11 arm to arm and 3 leg to leg).

- Ipsilateral spread: 10 patients (29%) (4 arm to leg and 6 leg to arm).

- Diagonal spread: 10 patients (29%) (4 arm to leg and 6 leg to arm).

Another factor they reported on was spontaneous spread of CRPS. This form of spread from a first to a second limb was seen in(25):

- Contralateral spread: 24 patients (63%) (11 arm to arm, and 13 leg to leg).

69

- Ipsilateral spread: 13 patients (34%) (8 arm to leg, and 5 leg to arm).

- Diagonal spread: 1 patient (3%).

Additionally, they observed that patients with ML-CRPS exhibited movement disorders, and those with this condition also experienced a longer duration of the disease(25).

In 2020, Eriksen and colleagues, reviewed a case of a patient with severe symptoms of CRPS affecting multiple limbs. The patients symptoms were resistant to treatments. The patient had undergone treatment with a spinal cord stimulator (SCS). The patient had some initial relief from the SCS, but unfortunately, the patients CRPS symptoms progressed, affecting all four limbs. The patient developed a complication with the SCS. One of the SCS leads had fractured and cause a recurrence of CRPS in the patients arm, which unfortunately had to be amputated due to the pain (26).

They concluded, when a patient with an SCS implant experiences a rapid increase in symptoms or the sudden stoppage of stimulation, it is crucial to consider mechanical issues as a possible cause(26).

70

TOTAL BODY CRPS(TB-CRPS)

In 2009, Doctor Schwartzman and colleagues, published an article, titled The Natural History of Complex Regional Pain Syndrome. In this article they addressed the patterns of pain spread. They found 35% of CRPS patients reported spread of symptoms to the whole body(TB-CRPS)(27).

In 92% of patients in their study reported spread of their pain to other body parts during the course of their disease(27).

They found contiguous spread developed in patients within one to two years, which is the most common form of spread during the first 10-years after the onset of the disease. Spread to other extremities during the course of the disease with no specific pattern of spread(27).

Spread of the disease into all extremities was seen in patients 15-years after the onset of CRPS(27).

In 2012, a study conducted by Doctor Schwartzman, focused on 2,500 patients with CRPS. Among them, 29 patients (39%) were found to have TB-CRPS(28).

71

In 2013, Edinger, et al., reported that CRPS is a syndrome which can spread from the initial injury site to encompass the total body in long standing cases(29).

SURGERY AS A CAUSE OF SPREAD IN CRPS

According to Dobritt and Hartrick, they reviewed a case of severe, chronic, bilateral CRPS following multiple laminectomies (30). They reported the bilateral damage to the sinuvertebral nerve from previous surgery or epidural adhesions could have caused CRPS on a peripheral basis in this patient(30).

In a patient with a known history of CRPS, Satteson, et al., reported there is a greater risk of CRPS spreading to a previously unaffected extremity after a new traumatic insult, such as a surgical procedure(31).

REFERRED PAIN IN CRPS

Many CRPS patients suffer from referred pain. This observed phenomenon of referred pain of CRPS can sometimes be mistaken for the spread of the disease. These are two separate issues that patients go through (1-3).

MULTIPLE LIMB-CRPS AND TOTAL BODY-CRPS SURVEY STUDY

In May 2024, I conducted a brief survey among Facebook users who were diagnosed with CRPS and experienced complications of spread of their CRPS symptoms to another limb or to their entire body. The survey included 48 participants, with 45 females and five males.

The participants reported that their CRPS symptoms had spread to other areas of their body, with the earliest occurrence happening, one month after the disease started, and the latest occurring up to 10-years after the first symptoms of CRPS appeared.

All 47 patients developed spread after onset of CRPS into the following:

- Two limbs: 14 patients(29%).
- Three limbs: 9 patients(19%).
- Four limbs(not total-body spread): 4 patients(8%).
- Total body(TB)(including other body parts): 21 patients(44%).

In addition, five patients developed internal organ spread; three patients developed spread after receiving a spinal cord stimulator(SCS) implant; two patients developed symptoms of spread in the lower back after an injury; and two patient developed spread into the orofacial area.

73

This small survey outcome represent only a fraction of the countless cases where patients have developed the spread of their CRPS symptoms to multiple limbs or their entire body.

CONCLUSION

Diagnosing and treating CRPS can be challenging due to its complexity. One of the main issues faced by CRPS patients is the potential spread of the syndrome. Coping with CRPS in a single limb can be incredibly tough and painful for individuals.

Unfortunately, some CRPS patients will experience spread of the disease from one limb to multiple limbs, total body spread, spread to the face, or develop internal organ involvement.

In some CRPS cases the development of spread is cause by the following:

- Spontaneous spread.
- Spread from a new injury.
- Spread from surgery.

In some instances, patients may experience disease progression spontaneously as a result of the disease's duration and absence of treatment.

Due to the spread of the disease, the patient's life becomes more complicated and distressing. It is crucial for the treating physician to recognize that CRPS can spread through various factors, and early detection and treatment are essential in stopping the progression of this relentless and agonizing syndrome.

Having CRPS in one limb is painful, unbearable, and unthinkable. Imagine having it in multiple limbs or total body with internal organ involvement.

It is unimaginable for those unfamiliar with CRPS to comprehend the immense suffering and agony endured by patients living with this condition. Whether it affects a single limb or multiple limbs, the constant sensation of being engulfed in flames on a daily basis for extended periods of time, ranging from one to thirty plus years or longer, is beyond comprehension. The relentless nature of this pain has the potential to drive anyone to the brink of insanity.

The medical community has yet to fully acknowledge the extent of CRPS spread and lacks understanding of the mechanisms behind its progression to other body parts, whether spontaneously or due to additional trauma or surgery.

It is crucial to conduct further research on the factors contributing to the spread of CRPS. This will help us better understand the condition and improve treatment outcomes for patients.

REFERENCES

1. Phillips EM. Complex Regional Pain Syndrome (CRPS): Learning About The Different Aspects of a Painful Syndrome: Volume I. Amazon Books. 2022. Chapter 5; 64-87.

2. Hooshmand H, Phillips, EM. Spread of complex regional pain syndrome (CRPS). 2009; 1-11. www.rsdrx.com and www.rsdinfo.com

3. Phillips EM. Complex Regional Pain Syndrome (CRPS): Learning About The Different Aspects of a Painful Syndrome: Volume I. Amazon Books. 2022. Chapter 6; 88-117.

4. Hooshmand H. Chronic Pain: Reflex Sympathetic Dystrophy: Prevention and Management. CRC Press, Boca Raton FL. 1993.

5. Veldman PH, Goris RJ. Multiple reflex sympathetic dystrophy. Which patients are at risk for developing a recurrence of reflex sympathetic dystrophy in the same or another limb? Pain 1996; 64: 463-466.

6. Kozin F, McCarty DJ, Sims J, et al. The reflex sympathetic dystrophy syndrome. I. Clinical and histologic studies: Evidence of bilaterality, response to corticosteroids and articular involvement. Am J Med. 1976; 60:321-331.

7. Radt P. Bilateral reflex neurovascular dystrophy following a neurosurgical procedure. Clinical picture and therapeutic problems of the syndrome. Confin Neurol 1968; 30:341-348.

8. Hooshmand H, Phillips EM. Various complications of complex regional pain syndrome (CRPS). www.rsdinfo.com and www.rsdrx.com Feb 16, 2016.

9. Schwartzman RJ, Popescu A. Reflex sympathetic dystrophy. Current Rheumatology Reports. 2002; 4(2):165-169.

10. Schwartzman RJ. Reflex sympathetic dystrophy. Handbook of Clinical Neurology. Spinal Cord Trauma, H.L. Frankel, editor. Elsevier Science Publisher B.V. 1992; 17: 121-136.

11. Hooshmand H, Hashmi H. Complex regional pain syndrome (CRPS, RSDS) diagnosis and therapy. A review of 824 patients. Pain Digest 1999; 9:1-24.

12. Hooshmand, H, Hashmi, M, Phillips, EM. Cryotherapy can cause permanent nerve damage: A case report. AJPM 2004;14: 2: 63-70.

13. Merskey H, Bogduk N. Classification of Chronic Pain Descriptions of Chronic Pain Syndromes and Definitions of Pain Terms. Task Force on Taxonomy of the International Association for the Study of Pain. Merskey, H. editor. IASP Press. Seattle 1994.

14. Dielissen PW, Claassen AT, Veldman PH, et al. Amputation for reflex sympathetic dystrophy. J Bone Joint Surg Br. 1995; 77: 270-273.

15. Veldman PH, Goris RJ. Surgery on extremities with reflex sympathetic dystrophy. Unfallchirurg 1995; 98: 45-48.

16. Schwartzman RJ, McLellan TL. Reflex sympathetic dystrophy. A review. Arch Neurol 1987; 44: 555-561.

17. Livingston WK. Pain mechanisms: A physiological interpretation of causalgia and its related states. In London, MacMillan 1943. (reprinted: Plenum Press, New York, 1976).

18. Phillips EM. Complex Regional Pain Syndrome (CRPS): Learning About The Different Aspects of a Painful Syndrome: Volume V. Amazon Books. 2024. Chapter 10; 179-207.

19. Veldman PH, Reynen HM, Arntz IE, et al. Signs and symptoms of reflex sympathetic dystrophy: prospective study of 829 patients. Lancet 1993; 342:1012-1016.

20. Maleki J, LeBel AA, Bennett GJ, Schwartzman RJ. Patterns of spread of complex regional pain syndrome, type I (reflex sympathetic dystrophy). Pain 2000; 88: 259-266.

21. Leriche R. The Surgery of Pain, Translated and edited by A. Young. Baltimore. Williams and Wilkins Company. 1939.

22. de Takats G. Causalgic states in peace and war. Journal of the American Medical Association. 1945; 7;128(10):699-704.

23. Greatorex F. Complex Regional Pain Syndrome, Type 1: Spread of symptoms and the involvement of the sympathetic nervous system (Doctoral dissertation, Murdoch University) 2002.

24. Khan EI, Scarlet P. Complex regional pain syndrome in all four limbs. European Journal of Anaesthesiology. 2007; 24(4):379-380.

25. van Rijn MA, Marinus J, Putter H, Bosselaar SR, Moseley GL, van Hilten JJ. Spreading of complex regional pain syndrome: not a random process. J Neural Transm (Vienna). 2011; 118: 1301-1309.

26. Eriksen LE, Terkelsen AJ, Sørensen JC, et al. Multiple limb involvement in a severe case of complex regional pain syndrome treated with spinal cord stimulation: a case report. A&A Practice. 2020; 1: 14(7):e01224.

27. Schwartzman RJ, Erwin KL, Alexander GM. The natural history of complex regional pain syndrome. The Clinical journal of pain. 2009; 1;25(4):273-280.

28. Schwartzman RJ. Systemic complications of complex regional pain syndrome. Neuroscience and Medicine. 2012; 25;3(03):225-242.

29. Edinger L, Schwartzman RJ, Ahmad A, et al. Objective sensory evaluation of the spread of complex regional pain syndrome. Pain Physician. 2013;16:581-591.

30. Dobritt DW, Hartrick CT. Reflex sympathetic dystrophy associated with multiple lumbar laminectomies. The Clinical journal of pain. 1986; 1;2(2):119-122.

31. Satteson ES, Harbour PW, Koman LA, et al. The risk of pain syndrome affecting a previously non-painful limb following trauma or surgery in patients with a history of complex regional pain syndrome. Scandinavian Journal of Pain. 2017;14(1):84-88.

CHAPTER 5

COMPLEX REGIONAL PAIN SYNDROME (CRPS) AND PREGNANCY

Eric M. Phillips

Abstract. Complex regional pain syndrome (CRPS) is a complex form of neuropathic pain, which has been reported in cases during pregnancy.

A limited amount of literature has been published over the past few decades regarding the topic of CRPS and pregnancy. This is an important topic to address for women who are in the reproductive age group and are considering to become pregnant while suffering from CRPS.

There are three important aspects of CRPS and pregnancy that should be acknowledged. In the reproductive age group, women with CRPS have the potential to become pregnant, and there are cases where CRPS can develop during pregnancy. Additionally, some patients with CRPS can experience a brief remission of their CRPS symptoms while pregnant.

Keywords. Complex regional pain syndrome (CRPS), CRPS and full-term pregnancy, pregnancy induced CRPS, and CRPS remission during pregnancy.

INTRODUCTION

According to my mentor the late Doctor Hooshmand, there is no contraindication for a CRPS patient to become pregnant. As for pregnancy-related CRPS, it may appear for the first time during pregnancy(1).

It is crucial to provide pregnant CRPS patients with information about the limited treatment options available during pregnancy, to ensure the safety of both the mother and the unborn baby.

To ensure a successful pregnancy and effectively manage CRPS, it is essential to involve a multidisciplinary team, including anesthesia, neonatology, obstetrics, and pain management. This collaboration should ideally start early in the pregnancy.

In this chapter I will discuss more about the important aspects of CRPS and pregnancy.

CRPS AND FULL-TERM PREGNANCY

From the research done by Doctor Hooshmand on the topic of CRPS and pregnancy, he would advise his pregnant CRPS patients to aim for a full-term delivery unless their pelvis was exceptionally small. This is because a C-section surgery can worsen CRPS symptoms. However, it is generally safe for CRPS patients to have a normal delivery, as long as the mother minimizes her intake of morphine and reduces or eliminates other medications that may result in fetal deformities. Specifically, medications like Fentanyl or Methadone should be avoided as they can be harmful to the baby(2).

PREGNANCY INDUCED CRPS

According to Doctor Hooshmand, CRPS may manifest itself for the first time during pregnancy(1).

In 1959, Doctors Curtis and Kincade, reported the first cases of pregnancy induced CRPS seen in three patients (3).

In 1999, Doctor Poncelet and colleagues, reviewed a series of nine cases of CRPS and pregnancy, and they also performed a review of the literature of (57 patients and 159 sites of CRPS) (4). They found that the hips was involved in 88%, the knee in 25%, and the ankle in 21% of cases, and the symptoms of CRPS had develop in the third trimester of pregnancy, between the 26th and the 34th weeks(4).

Additionally, it was determined that the only affected joints were those of the inferior limbs. A magnetic resonance imaging (MRI) was helpful for diagnosing, and they recommend that treatment should be non-aggressive (4).

In their study, they concluded that CRPS does not appear to affect the course of pregnancy(4).

In 2002, Zrigui, et al., reviewed a case of a 40-year-old woman who developed CRPS in her lower limbs during the fifth month of her third pregnancy (5). In addition, they reported that hips are the most common location for CRPS during pregnancy (5).

They also mention that during pregnancy, it is common for CRPS to be misdiagnosed or go unnoticed. The symptoms of CRPS can appear in the initial pregnancy, or in subsequent pregnancies(5).

In 2003, Sergent, et al, reported on a case of a patient who developed symptoms of CRPS in both ankles in her first trimester of pregnancy. They report that CRPS symptoms during pregnancy is usually seen in the hip (nine times out of 10), and fracture is the major risk of developing CRPS. They also report that symptoms of CRPS start in the third trimester of pregnancy(6).

In 2007, Karakoç, and colleagues, reviewed a case of a 25-year-old pregnant woman at 30 weeks gestation who had developed right foot and ankle pain. She had no prior history of trauma before her pregnancy (7). In their report they described the patient had developed symptoms of CRPS in her right foot and ankle during her pregnancy(7).

In their opinion, the factors contributing to CRPS during pregnancy have not been fully explained. They explain that during pregnancy some patients may develop significant weight gain, hyperlordosis, hypertriglyceridemia, and vascular stasis induced by the compression on the inferior vena cava (IVC) which may be risk factors for CRPS (7).

Their study acknowledges that CRPS may be a cause of acute foot and ankle pain during pregnancy. It is important to recognize this uncommon source of pain during pregnancy to avoid delays or incorrect diagnosis, during pregnancy(7).

In 2019, Baykara and colleagues documented a case involving a 28-year-old patient who was 32 weeks pregnant and had given birth during her 36th week. Additionally, the patient was diagnosed with CRPS (8). They suggest the diagnosis of CRPS should be taken into consideration when the present of lower extremity pain is report during pregnancy(8).

CRPS REMISSION DURING PREGNANCY

Pregnancy has been associated with temporary remission of CRPS symptoms, although the duration varies. While the remission is usually brief, there have been instances where it can persist for a few months following childbirth.

According to Doctor Hooshmand, as the pregnant CRPS patient goes into the later stages of pregnancy, the baby naturally supplies the mother with essential hormones like endorphins, estrogen, and growth hormones, which can greatly alleviate the symptoms of CRPS. This often leads to significant improvement with her symptoms of CRPS. However, after giving birth, the mother is no longer receiving these hormones, causing the pain associated with CRPS to resurface(2).

In 2020, Albano et al., conducted a review of a case involving a 38-year-old woman who was at 38 weeks and 2 days of pregnancy. At the age of 16, the patient developed CRPS. She went through several spinal surgeries, one of which involved the placement of a spinal cord stimulator (SCS) implant. Additionally, she received Ketamine infusions every six months until she became pregnant. Her CRPS symptoms went into remission when she became pregnant (9). The patient's remission was attributed to the elevated levels of progesterone(a steroid hormone) during pregnancy (9).

CRPS AND PREGNANCY SURVEY STUDY

In March 2024, I carried out a short survey study involving 11 female Facebook users who had been diagnosed with CRPS and had gone through pregnancy while dealing with their condition.

Among the 11 participants, only six patients achieved remission while they were pregnant. The remaining five patients did not experience remission during their pregnancy. Regrettably, one patient suffered two miscarriages, another patient lost her baby at 37 weeks, and a third patient lost her baby due to the medication she was taking for her CRPS treatment.

In this survey study, some patients did experience a brief remission during pregnancy, while others did not.

- One patient had increased pain during pregnancy.
- Two patients had no changes in their pain during pregnancy.

- One patient had reduced symptoms during all four of her pregnancies.
- One patient had two pregnancies and two remissions.
- One patient had a remission during pregnancy, but her symptoms came back after giving birth.
- One patient had two pregnancies and only one remission.
- One patient had remission during pregnancy and it continued after giving birth and during breastfeeding for a few months.
- One patient had three pregnancies and two remissions.
- One patient had two pregnancies and no remissions.
- One patient had four pregnancies and only one remission during her third pregnancy.

This brief survey illustrates the impact of pregnancy on women in the reproductive age group who suffer from CRPS.

CONCLUSION

In the context of CRPS and pregnancy, patients can be divided into two categories. The first category includes CRPS patients who have the possibility of becoming pregnant, while the second category involves cases where CRPS can manifest during pregnancy.

It is crucial to educate CRPS patients of reproductive age about the limited treatment options available to them during pregnancy. In cases where a pregnant patient develops CRPS symptoms, it is essential to promptly diagnose and address their symptoms.

Some pregnant CRPS patients may experience a temporary relief or remission of their symptoms during pregnancy.

The management of CRPS symptoms becomes increasingly complex during pregnancy due to the need to prioritize the health of both the patient and her unborn child. Collaborating with a skilled multidisciplinary team is crucial in developing an effective strategy to support the CRPS patient throughout her pregnancy.

REFERENCES

1. Hooshmand H. RSD PUZZLE #7: RSD and Pregnancy. 1996; www.rsdrx.com.

2. Hooshmand H. RSD PUZZLE #141: Full-Term Pregnancy and RSD. 1997; www.rsdrx.com.

3. Curtiss Jr PH, Kincaid WE. Transitory demineralization of the hip in pregnancy: a report of three cases. JBJS. 1959;41:1327-1333.

4. Poncelet C, Perdu M, Levy-Weil F, et al. Reflex sympathetic dystrophy in pregnancy: Nine cases and a review of the literature. European Journal of Obstetrics & Gynecology and Reproductive Biology. 1999; 86: 55-63.

5. Zrigui J, Etaouil N, Mkinsi O. Reflex sympathetic dystrophy and pregnancy: A case report. Joint Bone Spine. 2002; 69: 342-344.

6. Sergent F, Mouroko D, Sellam R, et al. Algoneurodystrophie de la cheville au cours d'une grossesse: particularités et prise en charge thérapeutique [Reflex sympathetic dystrophy involving the ankle in pregnancy: characteristics and therapeutic management]. Gynecol Obstet Fertil. 2003; 31: 543-545. In French.

7. Karakoç M, Altındağ Ö, Neslihan S. Reflex sympathetic dystrophy syndrome of the ankle in pregnancy. Rheumatism. 2007;22:76-79.

8. Baykara RA, Tuzcu G, Karabacak P, et al. Foot-ankle involvement of complex regional pain syndrome associated with pregnancy. The European Research Journal. 2019;5:428-432.

9. Albano JL, Brothers JL, Landa S, et al. Cesarean section in a patient with complex regional pain syndrome. St. Joseph's University Medical Center Paterson, NJ. Society for Obstetric Anesthesia and Perinatology, Annual Meeting-Poster Abstract; 2020.

CHAPTER 6

ENDOCRINE SYSTEM DYSFUNCTION(ESD) IN COMPLEX REGIONAL PAIN SYNDROME (CRPS)

Eric M. Phillips

Abstract. Complex regional pain syndrome (CRPS) has a consequential impact on the endocrine system which can cause hormonal imbalance in some CRPS patients. The endocrine system dysfunction(ESD) seen in some cases of CRPS must be recognized by the treating physician, and it needs to be treated appropriately, to spare the patient from suffering from the added pain caused by the dysfunction of the endocrine system.

Keywords. Complex regional pain syndrome (CRPS), endocrine system, endocrine system dysfunction(ESD), hormonal imbalance, hypothyroidism, and low serum cortisol levels.

INTRODUCTION

Many complications arise during the progression of complex regional pain syndrome (CRPS). One such complication observed in certain CRPS patients is endocrine system dysfunction (ESD).

94

There have been limited reports published regarding the effects of ESD in patients with CRPS. It is crucial to identify the symptoms associated with ESD at an early stage, as this will assist in devising a treatment plan aimed at averting additional complications associated with ESD in patients with CRPS.

The medical community has to understand and recognize that the complications of ESD in CRPS patients are serious and they can create more issues for the patient over time.

In this chapter I will discuss more about the complications of ESD associated with CRPS.

THE ENDOCRINE SYSTEM

The severe pain of CRPS may cause notable disruptions in the endocrine system, resulting in hormonal imbalances.

In Doctor Hooshmand's 1993 textbook on reflex sympathetic dystrophy (RSD), he states that the brain is an endocrine gland that regulates behavior through hormone secretion (1). There are two types of cells in the brain. The nerves, and the glial cells protecting the nerves. Hormones are secreted by the nerves, while glial cells do not have this ability.

Endorphins, which are potent hormones, play a crucial role in controlling pain. Unlike endorphins, exorphins (e.g., Codeine, Demerol, Heroin, and Morphine) require significant amounts (10-20 nanograms or billionths of a gram) to be effective. Apart from pain relief, their actions differ completely(1).

ENDOCRINE SYSTEM DYSFUNCTION(ESD) IN CRPS

CRPS cases can display many different types of endocrine system dysfunction (ESD), such as the following:

- Adrenal insufficiency.
- Depression.
- Hormonal imbalances.
- Hypothyroidism.
- Low cortisol levels.

According to Buryanov and colleagues, endocrine dysfunction (ESD) in CRPS patients causes hormonal imbalances in the hypothalamic-pituitary-adrenal and hypothalamic-pituitary-gonadal systems (2).

Their research also found that women with CRPS had lower cortisol levels. In addition, they found that female CRPS patients had reduced androgenic(sex hormones) function of the adrenal cortex (2).

The research work by Doctor Schwartzman et al., reported that one third of CRPS patients suffer from Hypothyroidism and low serum cortisol levels in 38% of CRPS cases (3-5). Doctor Schwartzman also reported that 69% of patients described unusual fatigue and severe tiredness (3,6).

Ten out of the twenty-six patients in Doctor Schwartzman's study exhibited low baseline cortisol levels, with one patient also showing a low thyroid stimulating hormone (TSH) level (3,6).

The findings of his team's study reveal that a considerable number of CRPS patients exhibit low cortisol levels despite having normal adrenal function, indicating a malfunction in the hypothalamic-pituitary-adrenal (HPA) axis. A significant proportion of patients suffering from severe CRPS receive high doses of potent opioids for treatment(3,6).

Rhodin et al., reported that cessation of narcotics can help reverse endocrine system dysfunction (3,7).

HORMONE REPLACEMENT

Doctor Hooshmand, suggests that hormone replacement therapy can enhance cognitive functions by influencing the formation of excitatory synapses and NMDA regulation through estrogen in both male and female brains during development(8).

In his review of 824 CRPS patients a study conducted on female CRPS patients revealed that regardless of age, they tend to experience menopausal symptoms such as hot flashes and excessive sweating. (8). The study measured serum estrogen levels in 60 female CRPS patients, showing levels between 87 to 195 PG/ml, compared to the normal range of 100 to 395 PG/ml. Estrogen replacement therapy was found to be effective in improving cognitive function and reducing hyperhidrosis symptoms in these patients(8).

He also reported in his study that 43 patients received infusion pump therapy for CRPS, resulting in a notable decrease in serum estrogen and testosterone levels. Out of these, 41 patients needed hormone replacement therapy, leading to an average pain reduction of 1.7 (on a scale of 0-10), which reduced or cleared up the lower extremity edema(8).

CONCLUSION

Endocrine system dysfunction (ESD) is a common issue that affects many CRPS patients as their disease progresses. These dysfunctions result in problems with the adrenal gland, imbalance of hormones, decreased levels of cortisol, and affect the thyroid. These complications are legitimate and have the potential to create serious problems for many patients suffering from CRPS.

Recognizing the complications linked to ESD in CRPS patients is crucial. Early identification and treatment are essential in preventing additional pain for the patients. Further research on the impact of ESD on CRPS is necessary to enhance the patient's quality of life.

REFERENCES

1. Hooshmand H. Chronic pain: Reflex sympathetic dystrophy. Prevention and management. Boca Raton, CRC Press 1993.

2. Buryanov A, Kostrub A, Kotiuk V. Endocrine disorders in women with complex regional pain syndrome type I. Eur J Pain. 2017; 21(2):302-308.

3. Hooshmand H, Phillips EM. Various complications of complex regional pain syndrome (CRPS). 2016. www.rsdinfo.com and www.rsdrx.com.

4. Schwartzman RJ, Erwin KL, et al. "The natural history of complex regional pain syndrome," The Clinical Journal of Pain 2009; Vol. 25, No. 4, 273-280.

5. Schwartzman RJ, Ambady P. Tertiary Adrenal In-sufficiency in CRPS: Effects of Chronic Pain on the Hypothalamic-Pituitary-Adrenal Axis. Unpublished.

6. Schwartzman RJ. Systemic complications of complex regional pain syndrome. Neuroscience & Medicine. 2012; 3, 225-242.

7. Rhodin A, Stridsberg M, Gordh T. Opioid endocrinopathy: A clinical problem in patients with chronic pain and long-term oral opioid treatment. Clin J Pain. 2010; 26(5):374-380.

8. Hooshmand H, Hashmi H. Complex regional pain syndrome (CRPS, RSDS) diagnosis and therapy. A review of 824 patients. Pain Digest. 1999; 9: 1-24.

CHAPTER 7

ELECTRIC SHOCK PAIN(ESP) IN
COMPLEX REGIONAL PAIN SYNDROME (CRPS)

Eric M. Phillips

Abstract. There are many different symptoms associated with complex regional pain syndrome (CRPS). The following are the main symptoms used to help rendered a proper diagnosis of CRPS: Burning pain or an ice-cold pain in the extremity caused by a minor trauma or surgery, discoloration of the skin, swelling (edema) of the extremity, and hypersensitivity of the skin (allodynia). CRPS is characterized by a wide range of symptoms. One symptom often overlooked when diagnosing the disease is the excruciating electric shock pain (ESP) experienced by a majority of CRPS patients throughout the course of their disease.

The sudden electric shock pain(ESP) experienced by CRPS patients is an intense and unexpected sensation that exacerbates their overall pain.

Keywords. Complex regional pain syndrome (CRPS), electric shock pain(ESP), and symptoms of CRPS.

INTRODUCTION

Comprehending and addressing the signs and symptoms of complex regional pain syndrome(CRPS) can be intricate. Physicians typically recognize the standard symptoms of CRPS, but there is an overlooked symptom known as electric shock pain (ESP), which can be both intriguing and distressing for patients. It is important not to disregard or overlook this unwelcome and agonizing symptom when patients report experiencing it alongside their other CRPS symptoms.

For patients suffering from CRPS, ESP is a distressing symptom characterized by recurring bouts of agonizing, pain that can occur at any time during the day or night. Like other symptoms of CRPS, ESP does not give the patient a warning sign when it will strike.

In this chapter I will discuss more about the effects of the painful symptom of ESP seen in CRPS cases.

ELECTRIC SHOCK PAIN SYMPTOMS IN CRPS

According to my mentor the late Doctor Hooshmand, he explains that ESP symptoms in CRPS are a result of electric shocks that occur when damaged nerve fibers come into contact with each other. Normally, nerve fibers are protected by a fatty sheath called "myelin". However, if an injury occurs and damages the adjacent nerve fibers, the insulating sheath is also affected. This leads to the spread of electrical current in the nerve fiber, causing irritation to the neighboring damaged nerve fibers (1).

Over time, the combined impact of nerve damage and irritation leads to a sudden electrical discharge, creating a sensation similar to an electric shock. In severe cases, this shock can briefly affect the nerves controlling posture and balance, causing the patient to potentially fall to the ground either partially or completely(1).

In CRPS, as the disease progresses, this particular symptom, along with other symptoms of CRPS, intensifies and becomes more noticeable. The worsening of the disease, caused by inflammation and swelling, contributes to the increased severity of this symptom. The occurrence of falling attacks is typically observed during the later stages (3rd and 4th) of the disease (1).

CRPS Type II (causalgia), which refers to the causalgic form of reflex sympathetic dystrophy(RSD), points to the fact that in causalgia there is ectopic and ephaptic nerve damage bypassing the synaptic transmission of electric current in nerve fibers between the adjacent damaged smaller and larger myelinated nerves (2-10).

Chang and colleagues, have described CRPS pain as often feeling like a burning sensation or being similar to repeated electrical shocks(11).

Lunden, et al., explain that spontaneous ongoing pain refers to the constant pain experienced by the patient, independent of any external stimuli. On the other hand, paroxysmal pain is characterized by sudden bursts of pain within the affected area, unrelated to any specific trigger. These bursts are often described as electric shocks(12).

In 2023, a study by Cruz and colleagues, detailed the case of a 40-year-old woman who suffered a right wrist injury requiring emergency surgery on the median nerve. Two months after the procedure, she was diagnosed with CRPS and experienced intense pain rated at a 10 on the pain scale during her initial assessment. She described symptoms including allodynia, burning pain, electric shock pain (ESP), and hyperalgesia(13).

ANTICONVULSANTS TREATMENT FOR
ELECTRIC SHOCK PAIN(ESP) IN CRPS

According to Doctor Hooshmand, treatment with anticonvulsants is helpful in CRPS for two types of symptoms(14):

- In patients who suffer from spinal cord sensitization leading to myoclonic and akinetic attacks.

- In patients who suffer from ephaptic or neuroma type of nerve damage characterized by stabbing, electric shock pain, or jerking type of pain secondary to damage to the nerve fibres.

In these types of cases, anticonvulsants, especially Tegretol (non-generic), Depakene, Gabapentin, and Klonopin (non-generic), are quite effective(14).

To effectively manage the ephaptic CRPS, a combination of effective anticonvulsants, antidepressants, and analgesics is recommended. Clonazepam has proven to be highly effective in controlling myoclonic jerks, and providing relief for patients(14).

MY PERSNOAL EXPERINCE WITH ELECTRIC SHOCK PAIN(ESP)

My personal experience with electric shock pain (ESP) started 38-years ago when I was involved in a car accident. During my accident I was a passenger in the car and fortunately or unfortunately, I saw the accident coming, so I had braced my left foot into the car's floorboard in an attempt to lessen the impact of the accident(big mistake!).

As the crash occurred, I experienced a sudden surge of an electric shock pain(ESP) that shot up from my left foot to my lower back. The electrical shock ("jolt" as I call it) I felt during the impact of the accident marked the beginning of a lifelong struggle with the aftermath of the accident, something entirely new to me.

The electric shock pain(ESP) I experienced during my accident was something which I had never felt before in my young 20-years of life at that time.

This accident and the electric shock pain that I felt that night would eventually lead me to a diagnosis of CRPS two years after my accident. During my 20-plus years with my former leg as I call it(since I am an amputee now), suffering and dealing with the unrelenting pain of CRPS, I had experienced years of torture with these agonizing episodes of ESP.

These ESP would interrupt my daily living. I would get these agonizing ESP during the day and especially at night, which I found to be the worst, because they would wake me up from a dead sleep. These ESP would be so violent that the jolts would lift my left leg right off the bed. I would feel these jolts go from my left foot straight up my left leg into my lower back, just like how it started during my car accident.

These ESP which I had experienced for over 20-plus-year were real. This unusual and complex symptom of CRPS is not totally understood by the medical community. Only another CRPS patient could understand and relate to this type of agonizing pain caused from the ESP due to CRPS.

In my case I feel that there is some type of a connection between the ESP, my CRPS and the herniated discs in my lower lumbar area, which I experienced during my car accident 38-years ago.

ELECTRIC SHOCK PAIN(ESP) IN CRPS SURVEY STUDY

In March 2024, I conducted a brief survey among Facebook users who were diagnosed with CRPS and had experienced symptoms of electric shock pain(ESP) since the onset of their CRPS. The survey included 45 participants, with 44 females and one male.

The participants in this study shared that they experienced the symptoms of ESP for a period spanning from two months to 41 years, starting from the onset and diagnosis of their CRPS.

The study found that all patients experienced ESP symptoms daily as their disease progressed. At night, some patients reported experiencing more intense ESP symptoms compared to their symptoms during the day.

Since the onset of their CRPS, the affected limb has exhibited symptoms of ESP. Among the 45 patients, only two experienced total body spread of CRPS that affected all four limbs, accompanied by symptoms of ESP.

The results of this survey only represent a small portion of the numerous cases in which patients have developed and experienced the symptom of ESP in their affected limb or entire body.

CONCLUSION

The symptom of electric shock pain (ESP) seen in CRPS cases is not rare. This painful symptom of CRPS affects many patients worldwide.

The symptom of ESP can start at the onset of the disease or it can manifest from a few months to a few years after the initial onset of CRPS.

109

Unfortunately, the symptoms of ESP are not fully recognized throughout the medical community as a serious symptom associated with CRPS. It is vital to understand and recognize that this complex symptom of CRPS is a painful and it creates more pain and discomfort for the patient.

In order to gain a more comprehensive understanding of how ESP affects the intensity of pain in individuals with CRPS, there is a need for further research into its mechanism.

REFERENCES

1. Hooshmand H. RSD Puzzle #79. Attacks of stabbing and electric shock pain In RSD patients. 1996. www.rsdinfo.com.

2. Phillips EM. Complex Regional Pain Syndrome (CRPS): Learning About The Different Aspects Of A Painful Syndrome: Volume I. Amazon Books. 2022. Chapter 10; 174-205.

3. Rasminsky M: Ectopic generation of impulses and cross - talk in spinal nerve roots of "dystrophic" mice. Ann Neurol. 1978; 3:351-357.

4. Seltzer Z, Devor M. Ephaptic transmission in chronically damaged peripheral nerves. Neurology. 1979; 29:1061-1064.

5. Merrington WR, Nathan PW. A study of post-ischaemic parasthesiae. J Neruol Neurosurg Psychiat. 1949; 12:1-18.

6. Ochoa JL, Torebjörk HE. Paraesthesiae from ectopic impulse generation in human sensory nerve. Brain. 1980; 103:835-853.

7. Ochoa JL, Torebjörk HE, Culp WJ, et al. Abnormal spontaneous activity in single sensory nerve fibers in humans. Muscle Nerve. 1982; 5:S74-77.

8. Torebjörk HE, Ochoa JL, McCann FV. Paresthesiae: Abnormal impulse generation in sensory nerve fibers in man. Acta Physiol Scand. 1979; 105: 518-520.

9. Devor M. Nerve patholophysiology and mechanisms of pain in causalgia. J Auton Nerv Syst. 1983; 7:371-384.

10. Devor M, Jänig W. Activation of myelinated afferents ending in a neuroma by stimulation of the sympathetic supply in the rat. Neurosci Letters. 1981; 24:43-47.

11. Chang C, McDonnell P, Gershwin ME. Complex regional pain syndrome - False hopes and miscommunications. Autoimmun Rev. 2019; 18(3):270-278.

12. Lunden LK, Kleggetveit IP, Schmelz M, et al. Cold allodynia is correlated to paroxysmal and evoked mechanical pain in complex regional pain syndrome (CRPS). Scand J Pain. 2022; 22(3):533-542.

13. Cruz AR, Sales FR, Maldonado F, Torres J, Cruz AR. Complex regional pain syndrome: is there a role for capsaicin? Cureus. 2023 Jan 25;15(1).

14. Hooshmand H, Hashmi H. Complex regional pain syndrome (CRPS, RSDS) diagnosis and therapy. A review of 824 patients. Pain Digest. 1999; 9: 1-24.

CHAPTER 8

PARESIS COMPLICATIONS IN
COMPLEX REGIONAL PAIN SYNDROME (CRPS)

Eric M. Phillips

Abstract. Paresis, a form of muscular weakness, is another symptom often overlooked in cases of complex regional pain syndrome (CRPS) and there is a lack of published data on the paresis-related complications reported by individuals with CRPS.

The development of paresis can vary, occurring within the first few months to a year after the initial onset of CRPS, and it can affect both the upper and lower extremities.

It is crucial for the treating physician to acknowledge the presence of paresis as a severe complication in CRPS patients. Timely identification and intervention are essential in preventing the affected extremity from becoming completely nonfunctional, thus preserving its use for the patient.

113

Keywords. Complex regional pain syndrome (CRPS), dystonia, idiopathic paralysis, muscular weakness, paresis, and spinal cord stimulators(SCS).

INTRODUCTION

According to my mentor, the late Doctor Hooshmand, weakness is an independent symptom of complex regional pain syndrome (CRPS) which can manifest with or without chronic fatigue(1).

CRPS patients experience muscle weakness not solely due to fatigue, but rather because the anterior horn cells and anterior lateral horn cells of the spinal cord are not coordinating properly and interfering with each other. In CRPS, the anterior lateral horn cells of the spinal cord release alpha adrenergic chemicals that lead to vasoconstriction, muscle spasms, and movement disorders(1).

The movement disorder can manifest as muscle weakness, spasms, tremors, dystonia, clumsiness, and difficulty coordinating rapid or repetitive movements. This can lead to limited mobility and weakness in the affected extremity(1).

114

The long-standing impairment of nerve and muscle function also causes gradual disuse atrophy of the extremity, thus pushing CRPS into stage III with atrophy and weakness of the affected extremity(1).

Doctor Peter Veldman and his team from the Netherlands, have observed that CRPS is often accompanied by paresis, a condition that may progress to paralysis. They refer to this symptom as pseudo-paralysis, as it is unrelated to nerve damage and can be identified through noticeable muscle contractions(2).

In this chapter I will discuss more about the complications of paresis seen in CRPS cases.

PARESIS COMPLICATIONS IN CRPS PATIENTS

According to Doctor Veldman, et al., they report paresis is one of the most frequent finding in CRPS (2,3). In these patients they complain of weakness of the affected CRPS limb. These patients have episodes of dropping objects out of their hands, difficulties of walking or lifting their foot. They also reports that this form of paralysis is not present at the onset of the disease and it cannot be attributed to nerve injury (3,4).

In a review of 829 CRPS patients, Doctor Veldman, and colleagues, reported that paresis has been seen as a complication in CRPS cases after the onset of the disease(4).

The below outlines the duration of paresis symptoms observed in cases of CRPS based on the elapsed time since the disease onset(4):

- From 0-2 months-92/94 patients=98%
- From 2-6 month-135/145 patients=93%
- From 6-12 months-122/134 patients=91%
- From one year or greater-151/156 patients=97%

Also, in 1995, Doctor Veldman, et al., reviewed a case of a 30-year old female who had sprained her left ankle while playing ice hockey in 1980. She developed cold-CRPS with symptoms of hyperpathia and progressive paresis. One year after her diagnosis of CRPS she developed a fixed dystonia. In 1985, her dystonia had spread into her upper extremities(5).

Birklein, et al., reported that around 80% of individuals with CRPS experience paresis weakness in their affected limbs which is caused by CRPS(6).

IDIOPATHIC PARALYSIS IN CRPS

In the opinion of Doctor Hooshmand, failure to treat CRPS aggressively or adequately, especially when the patient relies on assistive devices like a brace, cane, crutches, or a wheelchair, can lead to a rapid decline in CRPS weakness, ultimately preventing the patient from even standing. This so-called "idiopathic paralysis" is usually gradual and takes weeks or months to develop(1).

When it comes to the gradual development of idiopathic paralysis, there is an exception known as the "acute idiopathic paralysis" of CRPS. The sudden onset of paralysis in the lower extremities, which is acute in nature, can be attributed to two different types of treatments(1).

- Insertion of spinal cord stimulators(SCS).
- Insertion of indwelling catheter over the sympathetic chain of ganglia in the paraspinal region in the lumbar spine region.

Acute idiopathic paralysis is most frequently observed in patients who undergo SCS implantation in the spinal canal, affecting approximately 25% of patients. When the SCS is placed in an area of CRPS inflammation, the foreign body effect of the SCS can lead to a sudden worsening of muscle weakness and clumsiness, ultimately resulting in paralysis in the lower limbs(1).

When the insertion of SCS leads to such a phenomenon in a chronic pain patient, it is crucial to understand that the condition indicates a relatively severe CRPS, necessitating the immediate removal of the SCS(1).

A less common occurrence that has been increasingly observed in recent years involves inserting catheters into the epidural space or sympathetic ganglia chain area to avoid repeated needling for sympathetic nerve block in SCS patients. However, this is not as common among SCS patients(1).

It is crucial to promptly remove the catheter if paralysis occurs, rather than leaving it in overnight. Failure to remove the catheter for several days can lead to urinary and fecal incontinence in patients(1).

CONCLUSION

Paresis, a symptom observed in CRPS patients, poses a significant complication during the progression of the disease. Unfortunately, a majority of physicians treating CRPS patients do not fully acknowledge or understand how this complication affects CRPS patients.

Recognizing the symptom of paresis in CRPS patients is crucial as it is often neglected. Early treatment for paresis symptoms in CRPS is essential to avoid long-term complications for the patient.

Increasing awareness is essential to help both the medical community and CRPS patients understand the serious complications caused by symptoms of paresis due to CRPS.

REFERENCES

1. Hooshmand H. RSD PUZZLE #16. Fatigue, weakness, and "idiopathic paralysis." 1996; www.rsdinfo.com.

2. Veldman PH, Vingerhoets DM, Goris RJ. Pseudo-paralysis in reflex sympathetic dystrophy. A single fiber EMG study. CLINICAL ASPECTS OF REFLEX SYMPATHETIC DYSTROPHY. 1995. Chapter 8: 97-105.

3. Hooshmand H, Phillips EM. Various complications of complex regional pain syndrome (CRPS). 2016. www.rsdinfo.com and www.rsdrx.com.

4. Veldman PH, Reynen HM, Arntz IE, et al. Signs and symptoms of reflex sympathetic dystrophy: prospective study of 829 patients. Lancet. 1993; 342:1012-1016.

5. Veldman PH, Horstink MW, Goris RJ. Botulinum toxin does not relieve dystonia In patients with reflex sympathetic dystrophy. An argument for a muscular origin of the spasms? In: CLINICAL ASPECTS OF REFLEX SYMPATHETIC DYSTROPHY. 1995; Chapter 11: 131-138.

6. Birklein F, Riedl B, Sieweke N, et al. Neurological findings in complex regional pain syndromes--analysis of 145 cases. Acta Neurol Scand. 2000; 101(4):262-269.

CHAPTER 9

INTERNAL ORGAN COMPLICATIONS IN
COMPLEX REGIONAL PAIN SYNDROME (CRPS)

Eric M. Phillips

Abstract. The long-term consequences of complex regional pain syndrome (CRPS) include the spread of the disease to other body parts, and into the internal organs (visceral pain).

The painful internal organ complications experienced by patients with CRPS are a distressing aspect of the disease. Most doctors who treat CRPS are unaware that the condition can spread to other limbs and even affect internal organs.

The recognition and comprehension of this complex complication seen in certain CRPS patients is of utmost importance for the treating physician. Identifying the signs and symptoms of spread into the internal organs early is key to creating an effective treatment plan.

121

It is disappointing, that there is a lack of published data regarding internal organ-CRPS. Because of the complex complications that can arise from CRPS spreading internally, it is important to understand and recognize this serious subcomponent of CRPS.

Keywords. Complex regional pain syndrome (CRPS), internal organ-CRPS, and spread of CRPS.

INTRODUCTION

Another complication of complex regional pain syndrome (CRPS) is spread of the disease into internal organs. Doctors Hooshmand, Schwartzman, and Veldman are just few of a handful of doctors who have reported cases of CRPS affecting the internal organs in CRPS patients (1-4).

According to the late Doctor Robert J. Schwartzman, CRPS may also involve internal organs such as the GI tract. Approximately five percent of CRPS patients experience early satiety, bloating, nausea, and vomiting, which is considered to be a part of the clinical manifestations of gastroparesis, according to early evidence (5).

Doctor Schwartzman also reported that during the first five years of the disease, 47% of patients reported internal organ pain, and after 15-years after onset of CRPS, the percentage increased to 62%(4).

It's not uncommon for CRPS to spread to the internal organs, resulting in numerous complications and more pain for the patient. In this chapter, I will discuss more about the complications associated with internal organ-CRPS.

INTERNAL ORGAN SPREAD IN CRPS

CRPS invariably involves the internal organs. Usually, the skin surface is cold at the expense of increased circulation to the internal organs. This increased circulation can cause osteoporosis, fractures of bone, abdominal cramps and diarrhea, disturbance of absorption of foods with resultant weight loss, water retention with aggravation of premenstrual headaches and depression, persistent nausea, and vomiting, as well as severe vascular headaches mistaken for "cluster headache" (1,2).

In addition, CRPS can cause the complication of intractable hypertension which responds best to alpha I blockers (Dibenzyline, Hytrin, or Clonodine). CRPS can cause attacks of irregular or fast heart-beat, chest pain, coronary artery spasm (angina), as well as disturbance of function of other internal organs (1,2).

A few other examples are frequency and urgency of urination, respiratory disturbance such as dyspnea and apneic attacks, and attacks of severe abdominal pain (1,2).

Attacks of swelling of the internal organs complicated by intermittent constriction of the blood vessels to different organs can result in chest pain, attacks of sharp central pain (stabbing severe pain in the chest or abdomen), and changes in the patient's voice (suddenly developing a temporary "chipmunk" type of voice change). The sharp, stabbing, central pain can be helped with treatment with medications such as anticonvulsant (Tegretol or Neurontin) (1,2).

The internal organs complication may become aggravated by the traumatic effect of sympathetic nerve blocks. One such complication is accidental trauma to the kidney with resultant hematuria (blood in urine) and aggravation of hypertension (1,2).

Because of the above complex phenomenon, in CRPS the sympathetic nerves follow the path of the blood vessels rather than somatic nerve roots resulting thermotomal rather than dermatomal sensory nerve distribution (mistaken for hysterical sensory loss) may cause a complex clinical picture that baffles the clinician and forces the clinician to blame the patient as being hysterical, hypochondriac, and blaming the serious warning signs of CRPS complications as "functional and not organic"(1,2).

The end result is the deadly phrase **"it is all in your head"** which practically almost all CRPS patients have heard and had to deal with in the course of their treatment. The patient's symptoms and signs are real and they are not a figment of their imagination. The treating physician needs to take the time to learn and understand that the sympathetic system is complex, bilateral, and diffuse (1,2).

Doctor Schwartzman and colleagues, conducted a study in 2009, that analyzed 270 patients with CRPS and discovered that gastrointestinal (GI) complications were the most common internal organ complication among CRPS patients (4).

The following symptoms were reported by the patients in this study (4):

- Constipation (41%).
- Dysphagia(difficulty swallowing) (18%).
- Indigestion (18.5%).
- Intermittent diarrhea (18.5%).

- Irritable bowel syndrome (IBS) (17%).
- Nausea (23.3%).
- Vomiting (11.5%).

Doctor Schwartzman, states that almost all organ systems are involved during the course of CRPS(5).

AFFECTED INTERNAL ORGANS IN CRPS

After the onset of the disease, CRPS can spread to affect the following internal organs:

- Bladder.
- Cardiac system.
- G.I. system(gastroparesis, and reflux).
- Kidney.
- Lungs(low lung volume, and respiratory complications).
- Stomach.

MY PERSONAL EXPERIENCE WITH INTERNAL ORGAN-CRPS

During my tenth year of living with CRPS, I experienced an internal spread of the disease that affected the upper left side of my stomach near my rib cage. Throughout the years, I have had episodes of neuroinflammation in this particular area due to the spread of my CRPS.

The diagnosis of this spread into my stomach region was confirmed through a clinical examination and further supported by the use of infrared thermal imaging (ITI) performed by Doctor Hooshmand. Utilizing ITI proved to be beneficial in precisely identifying the internally affected area. The data obtained from the ITI played a crucial role in formulating a treatment plan aimed at reducing the internal neuroinflammation caused by the CRPS.

To address my internal organ CRPS symptoms, Doctor Hooshmand suggested implementing a treatment plan incorporating the use of IV Mannitol to mitigate the neuroinflammation occurring in my internal organs.

The treatment consisted of a dose of 100gm Mannitol in 500cc D5W (dextrose 5% in water). The course of treatment was conducted over a nine-week period.

- Three time a week for three weeks.
- Twice a week for three weeks.
- Once a week for three weeks.

127

The results were excellent. The Mannitol treatment had reduced my internal neuroinflammation by 90%.

A follow-up ITI was performed nine weeks after completing the treatment. The ITI proved to be highly beneficial in demonstrating the decrease in neuroinflammation of the internal organs caused by CRPS. Additionally, it highlighted the significant advantages of I.V. Mannitol treatment in effectively managing CRPS.

Mannitol is an inert sugar that acts as a selective strong diuretic, which can help reduce intracellular water retention.

It has proven that Mannitol is an effective and safe treatment option for patients, providing relief from the symptoms of neuroinflammation associated with CRPS.

INTERNAL ORGAN-CRPS SURVEY STUDY

In June 2024, I conducted a brief survey among Facebook users who were diagnosed with CRPS and had experienced symptoms of CRPS spread into their internal organs since the onset of their CRPS. The survey included 40 participants, with 38 females and two males.

The participants in this study shared that they experienced the symptoms of spread into their internal organs for a period spanning from one year to 14 years, starting from the onset and diagnosis of their CRPS.

The study found that all patients experienced spread of CRPS symptoms into the following internal organ systems:

- Bladder: 18 patients.
- Cardiac system: 11 patients.
- Colon: 1 patient.
- G.I. system: 31 patients.
- Kidney: 10 patients.
- Liver: 1 patient.
- Lungs: 3 patients.
- Pancreas (Exocrine pancreatic insufficiency (EPI)): 2 patients.

The results of this survey only represent a small portion of the numerous cases in which patients have developed and experienced the symptom of spread of CRPS into their internal organs.

CONCLUSION

The effects of CRPS are not restricted to the limbs after an injury or surgery. Unfortunately, during the course of the disease, the symptoms of CRPS can spread to other limbs and it can also affect the internal organs. The spread of this disease can occur spontaneously or over time.

In some cases of CRPS, the patient will experience spread of the disease from one limb to another, whole body spread, spread to the face, or develop internal organ involvement(1).

The spread of CRPS to another limb or internally is a genuine symptom of the disease, and it requires significant attention from the medical community treating CRPS patients.

To assist both the medical community and CRPS patients in understanding the serious complications caused by the spread of CRPS into internal organs, it is essential to raise awareness about this complex complication seen among many CRPS patients worldwide.

REFERENCES

1. Phillips EM. Complex Regional Pain Syndrome (CRPS): Learning About The Different Aspects of a Painful Syndrome: Volume I. Amazon Books. 2022. Chapter 5; 64-87.

2. Hooshmand H, Phillips EM. Various complications of complex regional pain syndrome (CRPS). 2016. www.rsdinfo.com and www.rsdrx.com.

3. Veldman PH, Reynen HM, Arntz IE, et al. Signs and symptoms of reflex sympathetic dystrophy: prospective study of 829 patients. Lancet. 1993; 342:1012-1016.

4. Schwartzman RJ, Erwin KL, et al. "The natural history of complex regional pain syndrome," The Clinical Journal of Pain 2009, Vol. 25, No. 4, 273-280.

5. Schwartzman RJ. Systemic complications of complex regional pain syndrome. Neuroscience & Medicine 2012, 3, 225-242.

CHAPTER 10

THE NAME CHANGE: WHAT SHOULD WE CALL IT?

CAUSALGIA, RSD, CRPS, OR SOMETHING NEW?

Eric M. Phillips

Abstract. The medical condition, commonly referred to as complex regional pain syndrome (CRPS), has been well documented throughout medical history. Unfortunately, this condition has been associated with multiple names since it was first documented in medical literature centuries ago.

There are several names associated with this condition, including causalgia, Sudeck's atrophy, reflex dystrophy, reflex neurovascular dystrophy (RND), shoulder-hand-syndrome, algodystrophy, reflex sympathetic dystrophy (RSD), or complex regional pain syndrome (CRPS). The name we give to this condition should not affect the significance of the extensive history of this condition.

132

Throughout the years, the name may have undergone alterations, but ultimately, the patient's pain remains unchanged. Increasing education in this area should be a top priority for the medical community. Young medical students must fully grasp the concept that regardless of the condition's name, the primary concern is the patient's suffering. They require an accurate diagnosis and an effective treatment plan to alleviate their pain.

Keywords. Causalgia, complex regional pain syndrome (CRPS), CRPS type I and II, chronic fatigue syndrome (CFS), fibromyalgia (FM), myofascial syndrome (MFS), and reflex sympathetic dystrophy(RSD).

INTRODUCTION

The term of complex regional pain syndrome (CRPS) was first introduced in 1994, by a consensus group at the International Association for the Study of Pain (IASP). The umbrella term of CRPS was officially agreed upon in 1995, at a medical conference in Orlando, Florida. The consensus group changed the terms of RSD to CRPS-type I and causalgia to CRPS type II.

This new term of CRPS was coined to replace the terms of causalgia which was first coined by Doctor Silas Weir Mitchell, in 1864(1), and reflex sympathetic dystrophy (RSD) which was first coined by Doctor James Evans from Boston Massachusetts in 1946(2).

We have been using the term CRPS to describe the painful condition previously known as RSD for the past 30 years. The medical and RSD communities have weighed the pros and cons of this name change, which has made the diagnosis and treatment plan more complex for both the treating physician and the patient.

According to Doctor Forest Tennant, he believes that renaming the terms causalgia and RSD to CRPS was meant to improve pain relief for patients suffering with this agonizing syndrome. However, this well-intentioned name change has resulted in unintended consequences. Moreover, one could argue that the renaming has been counterproductive(3).

Doctor Tennant advises removing the term CRPS. In his view, it reduces the severity of this severe condition, and the use of the term CRPS can actually hinder some patients from obtaining the necessary treatment(3).

Personally, living with RSD for the past 38 years, I have to agree with Doctor Tennant's view on the name change of this painful syndrome to CRPS. From my perspective, it would have been better to keep the term

134

RSD unchanged. This is because the term CRPS is often associated with various other painful syndromes, such as fibromyalgia (FM), chronic fatigue syndrome (CFS), myofascial syndrome (MFS), and many others.

By combining CRPS with other painful conditions, the medical community becomes confused, leading to multiple factors for the patient, such as delays in diagnosis, or receiving proper treatment.

In this chapter I will discuss more about how changing the term of RSD to CRPS affects both the medical and RSD communities.

THE DEFINITIONS OF CAUSALGIA, RSD, AND CRPS

Causalgia is characterized as a condition where pain persists after damage to a peripheral nerve has occurred.

In 1986, the International Association for the Study of Pain (IASP) described RSD as "persistent pain in a limb following injury, possibly a fracture, without major nerve involvement, accompanied by sympathetic hyperactivity" (4).

The definition of CRPS is a chronic pain disorder characterized by prolonged pain and inflammation in a particular part of the body, typically affecting the arm, hand, foot, or leg. It can develop from a minor trauma or a surgical procedure.

According to Doctor Geoffrey Schott, the clinical characteristics of RSD differ from those commonly associated with central or peripheral autonomic system diseases. In addition, RSD can occur in limbs that have undergone sympathectomy (5).

HISTORY OF CRPS

For many centuries there has been many reported cases written in medical literature reporting on the condition we now call complex regional pain syndrome (CRPS).

The earliest account of this painful condition was first reported and documented by Doctor Ambroise Paré, a French barber-surgeon. Doctor Paré was one of the first to describe what is now called CRPS, through his account of the persistent pain that King Charles IX had suffered from in the 16th century (6-8).

In the late 1700's, British surgeon Sir Pervcivall Pott, recognized burning pain and atrophy in injured extremities (6,8,9).

In 1813, Doctor Alexander Denmark reported a single case of a soldier who had an amputation due to burning pain (6,8-11). In 1838, Doctor James Hamilton had seen some cases in which his patients had symptoms of causalgia which resulted from accidental nerve injuries (6,8,12).

Early in 1864, Doctor James Paget had patients who had symptoms of constant warmth in their limb after nerve injury (6,8,13). Also, in 1864, Doctor Silas Weir Mitchell the father of American neurology gave the description of causalgia in his classic article Gunshot Wounds and Other Injuries of Nerves, but it was not until 1867 when he coined the term of causalgia from the Greek words, "Kausos"(καυσός) (heat) and "algos" (ἄλγος)(pain) to describe this syndrome (1,6,8).

Below are the dates and other names that have been associated with this painful syndrome:

- In 1900, Doctor Paul Sudek named it Acute bone atrophy(6,14).
- In 1901, Doctor Max Nonne* coined the term Sudeck's Atrophy (6,15).
- In 1916, Doctor René Leriche coined the term Sympathetic Neurites (6,16).
- In 1937, Doctor Geza DeTakats named it Reflex Dystrophy(6,17).

- In 1946, Doctor James Evans coined the term Reflex Sympathetic Dystrophy Syndrome (RSDS), he also suggested doing a sympathetic nerve block, thinking that it might be useful for pain relief(2,6).
- In 1947, Doctor Otto Steinbrocker named it Reflex Neurovascular Dystrophy and Shoulder-Hand Syndrome(6,18).
- In 1986, Doctor William B. Hobbins coined the term Reflex Sympathetic Dysfunction (6,19).
- In 1994 Doctor Harold Merskey, et al., gave the disease the new official name of Complex Regional Pain Syndrome (CRPS) (6,20).

*Doctor Max Nonne, was a medical student of Doctor Paul Sudeck. He coined the term "Sudeck's atrophy" in 1901.

OTHER NAMES ASSOCIATED WITH CRPS

Since Doctor Mitchell's first description of this painful syndrome in the United States, there have been many other names giving to this complex and painful disease (6).

Below are just a few of the many names that have been associated with the disease we now call CRPS(6):

- Post-traumatic painful osteoporosis - R. Leriche-1923 (6,20).
- Reflex limb dystrophy - G. De Takats-1937 (6,17).
- Minor & major causalgia -J. Homans-1940 (6,21).
- Shoulder-hand syndrome- O. Steinbrocker-1947 (6,18).
- Algodystrophy - S. de Sèze-1954 (6,22).
- Causalgia minor - R.D. Patman-1973 (6,23).
- Algo-neuro-dystrophy - E.N. Glick-1973 (6,24).

CONTRIBUTIONS MADE THROUGHOUT THE HSITORY OF RSD

In the last 81 years, there have been many key significant contributions made in the field of RSD. These contributions have come from committed physicians who have dedicated their entire professional lives assisting patients suffering from this painful disease.

The following are a few significant contributions that have improved our understanding of RSD:

- In 1943, Doctor William K. Livingston described the vicious circle of pain in RSD(6,25).
- In 1948; Doctor Sydney Sunderland described the perpetuation of pain and RSD at the spinal cord level(6,26).

- In 1973, Doctor John J. Bonica emphasized how the three stages of RSD are different from each other(6,27).
- In 1990, Doctor Robert J. Schwartzman discovered movement disorders in Reflex Sympathetic Dystrophy (RSD)(6,28).
- In 1993; Doctor H. Hooshmand described the four stages of RSD and the bilateral nature of RSD (6,9).

GUIDELINES FOR CRPS

In 1994, the International Association for the Study of Pain (IASP) developed a set of guideline for what we now call CRPS. This new guideline consist of classifying the disease into two categories:

- CRPS- type-I (RSD).
- CRPS- type-II (causalgia).

The new guidelines set forth by the IASP task force consist of patients having the following:

- A noxious event.
- Abnormal sudomotor activity.
- Allodynia.
- Changes in skin blood flow.

140

- Chronic pain after an injury or surgery.
- Edema.
- Hyperalgesia.

This diagnosis is ruled out due to the presence of other conditions that could explain the extent of pain and dysfunction.

In 2003, a consensus workshop group of 35 physicians from seven different countries organized by the International Association for the Study of Pain (IASP) took place in Budapest, Hungary. The purpose of this workshop was to introduce the Budapest criteria, a set of revised clinical diagnostic criteria, that aim to improve the specificity of the original IASP diagnostic criteria for CRPS (29).

In 2016, the European Pain Federation task force introduced 17 standards for diagnosing and managing CRPS in Europe. These goals are achievable for most countries, and ambitious for a few countries, depending on their healthcare resources and structures(30).

They developed the following 17 standards in eight areas of care for CRPS patients(30):

- One standard in assessment.

141

- Three standards for care pathways.
- Two standards in diagnosis.
- Two standard on distress management.
- One standard in education and information.
- One standard in multidisciplinary care.
- Four standards in pain management.
- Three standards in physical rehabilitation.

According to Goebel, et al., some European countries have developed their own guidelines for CRPS treatment(30).

In 2018, the Royal College of Physicians (RCP) of England, updated the guidelines for the management of CRPS. This guideline was updated by a group of 28 physicians (31).

UPDATED GUIDELINES AND CRITERIA FOR RSD

Since the new term of CRPS was introduced over 30 years ago to replace the term of causalgia and RSD, there have been multiple guideline and criteria changes made in the United States and throughout Europe.

These guideline and criteria changes have caused some confusion among the medical community and the RSD community.

Over the past three decades, the medical community has made significant progress in establishing a guideline system for managing the painful disease we now call CRPS.

Having lived with this disease for more than 38 years and being actively involved in the RSD community for over 30 plus years, I strongly believe that a global guideline for RSD is essential, given that RSD is a worldwide syndrome impacting millions of individuals, it is crucial to establish a global guideline for RSD to address its challenges.

Having a basic universal standard for diagnosing and treating RSD is essential, benefiting medical professionals, RSD patients, and insurance providers worldwide.

DOCTOR HOOSHMAND'S GUIDELINE CRITERIA FOR RSD

Below is a guideline criteria which was created by my mentor the late Doctor Hooshang Hooshmand. I propose we call this new guideline the "Hooshmand Criteria for RSD."

The criteria outlined in this guideline can help diagnose patients experiencing symptoms of RSD following a minor injury or surgery. By following these guidelines, healthcare providers can create an effective treatment plan for the patient.

143

RSD is a syndrome with multiple manifestations which require the following minimal symptoms and signs for the condition to be called RSD (32,33).

- Pain: constant, burning pain, and in some forms at times during the course of the disease, stabbing type of pain (causalgic). The pain is relentless and is invariably accompanied by allodynia (even simple touch or breeze aggravating the pain) and hyperpathia (marked painful response to simple stimulation).

- Spasms in the blood vessels of the skin and muscles of the extremities. The spasms in the blood vessels result in a very cold extremity. The muscle spasms result in a tremor, and movement disorders such as dystonia, flexion spasm, weakness, clumsiness of the extremities, and a tendency to fall.

- RSD is accompanied by a certain degree of inflammation in practically all cases. This inflammation may be in the form of swelling (edema), skin rash (neurodermatitis), inflammatory changes of the skin color (mottled or purplish, bluish, or reddish or pale discolorations), a tendency for bleeding in the skin, skin becoming easily bruised, inflammation and swelling around the joints as well as in the joints (such as wrists, shoulders, knee, etc.)

144

which can be identified on MRI in later stages, and secondary freezing of the joints.

- The fourth component and prerequisite of diagnosis of RSD are insomnia, and emotional disturbance. The fact that the sympathetic sensory nerve fibers carrying the sympathetic pain and impulse up to the brain, terminate in the part of the brain called "limbic system." This limbic (marginal) system which is positioned between the old brain (brainstem) and the new brain (cerebral hemispheres) is mainly located over the temporal and frontal lobes of the brain. The disturbance of function of these parts of the brain results in insomnia, agitation, depression, irritability, and disturbance of judgment. Insomnia is an integral part of an untreated RSD case. So are problems of depression, irritability, and agitation.

So, the clinical diagnosis of RSD is based on the above four principles rather than simply excluding RSD and finding some other cause for the patient's pain(32,33).

Below are some of the symptoms associated with RSD which should be recognized during the diagnosis process (32,33):

- Burning pain in the extremities.

145

- Chronic pain after injury or surgery.
- Cold pain feeling in the extremities.
- Discoloration of the skin.
- Edema (swelling of the extremities).
- Hypersensitivity to touch.
- Limited range of motion.
- Muscle spasms.

A NEW TASK FORCE FOR RSD IS NEEDED

I propose the establishment of a new task force aimed at simplifying a universal basic guideline criteria for patients with RSD. This task force should consist of knowledgeable physicians well-versed in the signs and symptoms of RSD, alongside a group of RSD patients who have battled the disease for more than two to three decades. It is crucial to incorporate the perspectives of individuals experiencing the debilitating pain of RSD.

Perhaps, after three decades of adhering to the current guidelines and terminology for CRPS, it may be prudent to consider implementing a fresh set of guideline criteria and a new term that accurately reflects the impact on the sympathetic nervous system following minor trauma or surgical procedures.

CONCLUSION

Throughout the past century and a half, this disease has undergone several name changes at different points in time. As, I have mentioned in the past, you can call it XYZ, causalgia, RSD, or CRPS, it does not matter what name we call it. It's all the same for the patient. This is a condition that causes unwanted pain and suffering.

In my own perspective, I think it would have been better to maintain the term RSD, as CRPS is categorized alongside other painful syndromes such as fibromyalgia (FM), chronic fatigue syndrome (CFS), myofascial syndrome (MFS), and numerous other syndromes. Since the name changed from RSD to CRPS, which took place 30 years ago, some in the medical community have downplayed the excruciating pain experienced by those with RSD.

I propose to put forth a new term to describe this painful and unwanted pain syndrome. My suggestion would be to name it "sympathetic nerve dysfunction syndrome" (SNDS or SND). I am suggesting this new term because this disease occurs when the sympathetic nervous system

147

becomes traumatize and damaged, usually because of minor trauma or surgery to the affected extremity.

I have no objections to using the old terms of causalgia or RSD, as they both provide a clear explanation of the signs and symptoms of this painful syndrome. However, I personally feel that introducing the term CRPS was unnecessary for several reasons. It has caused confusion among the medical community, the insurance industry, and contributed to delays in diagnosing and treatment for many patients.

In this chapter, I discussed how CRPS is often associated with other conditions, such as FM, MFS, and CFS. However, it's unfair to label RSD patients with other conditions that are not related to the unrelenting pain of RSD.

We need to have a basic universal guideline that can be used worldwide as a standard for the diagnosis and treatment of RSD. A guideline which is helpful to both the medical and RSD communities, as well as for the insurance industry.

Doctor Goebel and his colleagues, mentioned in their report that while the European Pain Federation task force guidelines for CRPS may be attainable for most countries, they could be challenging for a few nations due to varying healthcare resources and structures(30). Regardless of these differences, implementing a universal global guideline for diagnosing and treating RSD patients would greatly benefit the millions worldwide enduring the constant pain of RSD.

It is crucial to increase awareness and education about the debilitating condition of RSD among medical students, and the medical community. Regardless of the name given to this syndrome, what truly matters is the daily suffering of the patients. They require accurate diagnosis and effective treatment to alleviate their pain and improve their quality of life.

REFERENCES

1. Mitchell SW, Morehouse GR, Keen WW. Gunshot Wounds and Other Injuries of Nerves. Philadelphia: Lippincott, 1864.

2. Evans JA. Reflex sympathetic dystrophy. The Surgical Clinics of North America. 1946; 26:780-790.

3. Tennant F. CRPS is a bad name for a painful disease. Pain News Network. September 6, 2022.

4. Merskey H, Bogduk N. Classification of chronic Pain Descriptions of Chronic Pain Syndromes and Definitions of Pain Terms. Task Force on Taxonomy of the International Association for the Study of Pain. Merskey, H. editor. IASP Press. Seattle 1994.

5. Schott GD. Reflex sympathetic dystrophy. Journal of Neurology, Neurosurgery & Psychiatry. 2001, 1;71(3):291-295.

6. Phillips EM. Complex Regional Pain Syndrome (CRPS): Learning About The Different Aspects of a Painful Syndrome: Volume I. Publisher: Amazon Books. 2022 Chapter 1: 5-18.

7. Paré A. Les Ouvres d' Ambroise Paré, King Charles IX. 10th Book, Chapter 41. Paris Gabriel Buon 1598: 401.

8. Hooshmand H, Phillips EM. Various complications of complex regional pain syndrome (CRPS). www.rsdinfo.com and www.rsdrx.com Feb 16, 2016.

9. Hooshmand H. Chronic Pain: Reflex Sympathetic Dystrophy: Prevention and Management. CRC Press, Boca Raton FL. 1993.

10. Denmark A. An example of symptoms resembling tic douloureux produced by a wound in the radial nerve. Med Chir Trans. 1819; 4:48.

11. Richards RL. Causalgia: a centennial review. Arch Neurol 1967; 16:339.

12. Hamilton, J. On some effects resulting from wounds of nerves. Dublin J Med Sc. 1838; 13: 38–55.

13. Paget J. Clinical lecture on some cases of local paralysis. Med Times Hosp Gaz. 1864; 1:331.

14. Sudeck P. Ueber die acute entzuendliche Knochenatrophie. Arch Klin Chir. 1900; 62:147-156. In German.

15. Nonne M. Üeber radiographisch nachweisbare akute und chronische "Knochenatrophie" (Sudeck) bei Nerven-Erkrankungen. Fortsch. Geb. Röntgenstr.1901-1902; 5: 293-297.

16. Leriche R: De la causalgie, envisagee comme une nevrite du sympathique et de son traitement Par la denudation et l'excision des plexus nerveus periarteriels. Presse Med. 1916; 24:178-80.

17. De Takats G. Reflex dystrophy of the extremities. Arch Surg. 1937; 34: 939- 956.

18. Steinbrocker, O. Annals of the Rheumatic Diseases. 1947; 6, 80.

19. Hobbins WB. Basic concepts of thermology and its application in the study of the sympathetic nervous system. Second Albert Memorial Symposium, Washington, D.C., 1986.

20. Leriche R. Des oblitérations artérielles hautes (oblitération de la terminaison de l'aorte) comme cause des insuffisances circulatoires des membres inférieurs. Bull Mém Soc Chir (Paris). 1923;49:1404-1406.

21. Homans J. Minor causalgia: a hyperesthetic neurovascular syndrome. New Eng J Med 1940;222:870-874.

22. de Sèze S, Ryckewaert A. Algo-dystrophies sympathiques du member supérieur. En: Maladies des os et des articulations. Paris, Flammarion.1954.

23. Patman RD, Thompson JE, Persson AV. Management of post-traumatic pain syndromes. Report of 113 cases. Ann Surg. 1973;177:780-787.

24. Glick EN. Reflex dystrophy (algoneurodystrophy): results of treatment by corticosteroids. Rheumatol Rehabil. 1973; 12(2):84-88.

25. Livingston WK. Pain Mechanisms: A Physiologic Interpretation of Causalgia and Its Related States. New York: Macmillan. 1943.

26. Sunderland S, Kelly M. The painful sequelae of injuries of peripheral nerves. Aust N Z J Surg. 1948; 18(2):75-118.

27. Bonica JJ. Causalgia and other reflex sympathetic dystrophies. Postgrad Med. 1973 May;53(6):143-148.

28. Schwartzman RJ, Kerrigan J. The movement disorder of reflex sympathetic dystrophy. Neurology. 40:57-61 1990.

29. Harden RN, Bruehl S, Stanton-Hicks M, Wilson PR. Proposed new diagnostic criteria for complex regional pain syndrome. Pain Med. 2007 May-Jun;8(4):326-31.

30. Goebel A, Barker C, Birklein F, Brunner F, et al. Standards for the diagnosis and management of complex regional pain syndrome: Results of a European Pain Federation task force. Eur J Pain. 2019; 23(4):641-651.

31. Henderson J. Updated guidelines on complex regional pain syndrome in adults. J Plast Reconstr Aesthet Surg. 2019; 72(1):1-3.

32. Phillips EM. Complex Regional Pain Syndrome (CRPS): Learning About The Different Aspects of a Painful Syndrome: Volume III. Publisher: Amazon Books. 2023; Chapter 3: 26-44.

33. Phillips EM. Complex Regional Pain Syndrome (CRPS): Learning About The Different Aspects of a Painful Syndrome: Volume II. Publisher: Amazon Books. 2022; Chapter 10: 188-200.

CRPS INFORMATION RESOURCE PAGE

CRPS education, and awareness are very important to patients and their family members. Through education, awareness, and research maybe someday we can find a cure for CRPS?

For more helpful information on CRPS, please visit The International RSD Foundation at: www.rsdinfo.com Authors e-mail: utopia33@prodigy.net

CRPS Awareness Month!

Please tell your family and friends that November is CRPS Awareness Month. It is important for us to celebrate CRPS Awareness Month, to help spread and promote more awareness, and provide more education about this painful disease.

Please Write A Book Review On Amazon!

It would mean a lot to me if you could take a moment to write a review about this book:

COMPLEX REGIONAL PAIN SYNDROME (CRPS): LEARNING ABOUT THE DIFFERENT ASPECTS OF A PAINFUL SYNDROME- Volume: VI

Thank you, Eric

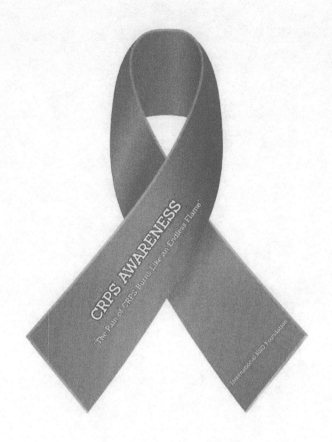

157

Made in the USA
Monee, IL
03 September 2024

64993336R00092